Oral Contraceptives & Breast Cancer

Committee on the Relationship Between
Oral Contraceptives and Breast Cancer

Institute of Medicine

Division of Health Promotion and Disease Prevention

NATIONAL ACADEMY PRESS
Washington, D.C. 1991

NATIONAL ACADEMY PRESS • 2101 Constitution Avenue, N.W. • Washington, D.C. 20418

NOTICE: The project that is the subject of this report was approved by the Governing Board of the National Research Council, whose members are drawn from the councils of the National Academy of Sciences, the National Academy of Engineering, and the Institute of Medicine. The members of the committee responsible for the report were chosen for their special competences and with regard for appropriate balance.

This report has been reviewed by a group other than the authors according to procedures approved by a Report Review Committee appointed by the members of the National Academy of Sciences, the National Academy of Engineering, and the Institute of Medicine.

The Institute of Medicine was chartered in 1970 by the National Academy of Sciences to enlist distinguished members of the appropriate professions in the examination of policy matters pertaining to the health of the public. In this, the Institute acts under both the Academy's 1863 congressional charter responsibility to be an adviser to the federal government and its own initiative in identifying issues of medical care, research, and education.

Support for this study was provided by the National Institute of Child Health and Human Development, pursuant to Contract No. N01-HD-9-2925.

Library of Congress Cataloging-in-Publication Data

Institute of Medicine (U.S.). Committee on the Relationship Between
   Oral Contraceptives and Breast Cancer.
   Oral contraceptives and breast cancer / Committee on the
   Relationship Between Oral Contraceptives and Breast Cancer,
   Institute of Medicine, Division of Health Promotion and Disease
   Prevention.
       p.   cm.
   Includes bibliographical references and index.
   ISBN 0-309-04493-6
   1. Breast—Cancer—Epidemiology—Congresses. 2. Oral
contraceptives—Side effects—Congresses. I. Title.
   [DNLM: 1. Breast Neoplasms—chemically induced.
   2. Contraceptives, Oral—adverse effects. 3. Risk Factors.   WP 870
   I575o]
   RA645.C3I57   1991
   616.99'449071—dc20
   DNLM/DLC
   for Library of Congress   91-19679
                                                               CIP

The serpent has been a symbol of long life, healing, and knowledge among almost all cultures and religions since the beginning of recorded history. The image adopted as a logotype by the Institute of Medicine is based on a relief carving from Ancient Greece, now held by the Staatlichemuseen in Berlin.

Committee on the Relationship Between Oral Contraceptives and Breast Cancer

*MAUREEN M. HENDERSON (*Chair*), Professor of Epidemiology and Medicine, University of Washington, and Head, Cancer Prevention Research Program, Fred Hutchinson Cancer Research Center, Seattle

LANETA J. DORFLINGER, Research Division, Office of Population, U.S. Agency for International Development, Washington, D.C.

JACK FISHMAN, President, IVAX Corporation, Miami, Florida

*HENRY W. FOSTER, JR., Dean, Meharry Medical College, Nashville, Tennessee

FRANK E. GUMP, Chief, Breast Service, Columbia-Presbyterian Medical Center, New York, New York

*SAMUEL HELLMAN, Dean, Division of Biological Sciences and The Pritzker School of Medicine, University of Chicago, Chicago, Illinois

*BARBARA S. HULKA, Kenan Professor and Chair, Department of Epidemiology, School of Public Health, University of North Carolina, Chapel Hill

DONALD R. MATTISON, Dean, Graduate School of Public Health, University of Pittsburgh, Pittsburgh, Pennsylvania

SUSAN A. R. McKAY, Professor, University of Wyoming School of Nursing, Laramie, Wyoming

---

*Member, Institute of Medicine.

---

iv

Preface

The Committee on the Relationship Between Oral Contraceptives and Breast Cancer was assembled in the fall of 1989 by the Division of Health Promotion and Disease Prevention of the Institute of Medicine (IOM) to examine the etiology of breast cancer as it relates to the use of oral contraceptives. The sponsor, the National Institute of Child Health and Human Development, asked the IOM committee to hold a conference to identify and highlight relevant issues, review policy options, offer suggestions for future research, and make recommendations for practicing physicians.

The questions addressed by the committee encompass clinical, personal, public health, and research matters. Are current oral contraceptive formulations safe? Will future pills be safer? What is the safest way to use them? Are they perfectly safe for some women but require judicious use by others? Do they increase breast cancer risk in women of all or only some ages? Could their widespread long-term use affect future nationwide breast cancer rates? Are there short-term markers of breast cancer that could be used to abbreviate epidemiological studies linking oral contraceptive use to subsequent clinical diagnoses of breast cancer? If short-term surrogate markers of breast cancer can be developed for this purpose, can they be used to unravel the causes of breast cancer? What must be done at a national level to ensure the safest personal and public health decisions about oral contraceptive use? Although some of these questions yielded to the committee's inquiry, others proved less tractable and will require further research.

Committee members were drawn from diverse scientific fields. They chose to assess the current state of knowledge of the beneficial or harmful influence of oral contraceptive use on breast cancer, patterns of use and changes in patterns of use, changes in formulations, biology of the breast, breast carcinogenesis, epidemiologic strategies, and animal and human research models and systems. A conference with invited speakers and prepared papers amplified the assessment. Four of the contributed papers, by Kathleen E. Malone, David B. Thomas, Diana B. Petitti, and David C. G. Skegg, are reproduced in this volume. Others are available from the National Technical Information Service.

The committee's interpretation and synthesis of the conference and contributed papers led to identification of gaps in current knowledge in many, if not all, of the dimensions noted above. This report recommends ways to begin to seek out information to fill those crucial gaps. In carrying out its task, the committee was ably supported and guided by its IOM staff colleagues.

MAUREEN M. HENDERSON, *Chair*
Committee on the Relationship Between Oral
Contraceptives and Breast Cancer

Contents

vii

Oral Contraceptives & Breast Cancer

Executive Summary

___

Oral contraceptives, which have been in use now for 30 years in the United States, are a highly effective and popular means of contraception. Data from 1988 indicate that at least 10.7 million American women currently use this method of contraception; 80 percent of 35-year-olds use, or have used, oral contraceptives. There are 17 different oral contraceptive formulations now available in the United States, which are marketed under 29 brand names.

Behind these impressive statistics are noteworthy trends: both the patterns of oral contraceptive use and the chemical formulation of the pills have been changing. The trends have been toward smaller and smaller doses of active hormones and increasing use by younger and younger women to prevent a first pregnancy, rather than to space successive pregnancies. Concomitant with the trend toward use at younger ages is the likelihood that today's young women will use oral contraceptives longer than previous, older users.

The introduction and dissemination of oral contraceptives in the United States have been superimposed on steadily rising breast cancer incidence rates. Breast cancer accounts for more new cases of cancer among American women than cancer of any other organ, and it has become more common through the twentieth century. One in nine women develops the disease sometime in her life, and 1 in 18 can expect to die from it.

Both pre- and postmenopausal endogenous hormones almost certainly play an important role in breast cancer, and their levels prob-

1

ably moderate the greater or lesser risk of women of different ages and with different reproductive histories. Therefore, it is biologically plausible that exogenous hormones, such as the synthetic estrogens and progestins found in oral contraceptives, have analogous effects. One should be prepared to find qualitatively and/or quantitatively different effects of exogenous hormones in older and younger women, and among women at any age with different reproductive histories.

Human studies of the effects of oral contraceptive use on breast cancer incidence have been complicated by the relatively short history of such use and a lack of stability of oral contraceptive formulations and usage patterns. Studies have collected and analyzed information only about relatively short-term exposures in women who started use as teenagers and about longer-term exposures among those who began to use the pill when they were in their 20s or early 30s. Both groups of women have had varied patterns of starting and stopping oral contraceptive use, and a majority have used two or more different formulations. (Oral contraceptives can vary in the types, amount, and ratios of hormones they contain.)

The utility of results of existing epidemiological studies in defining the relationship of oral contraceptives and breast cancer depends on whether they include exposures and follow-up intervals that are biologically feasible for identifying associations of both initiating and promoting events. Ideally, they should provide information about the dose, consistency, and duration of use, as well as the timing relative to reproductive physiological events (i.e., menarche, pregnancy, menopause) that perturb endogenous hormone levels.

There is considerable agreement about the consistency of results of the existing, prospective epidemiological studies. Thus far, the women in those studies have had no increases in breast cancer as they entered early postmenopausal years. Relatively few (about 10) additional years of follow-up are needed to determine whether the findings hold for later postmenopausal years. This follow-up, as well as a dedicated effort to prepare the results of existing cohort studies for pooled analysis, should be enough to confirm the existing consensus and put statistical limits on the upper bounds of measured safety with respect to the risk of breast cancer. There may also be sufficient data from this effort to determine whether oral contraceptive exposure of these virtually first users has had any impact in their postmenopausal years. The lack of an association between oral contraceptive use and postmenopausal breast cancer in these women would be an encouraging finding that will need to be confirmed among women who have long-term exposure from an early age. Studies of the impact of oral contraceptive use on postmenopausal breast cancer rates are imperative, because the majority of all breast cancer cases occur in the postmenopausal years.

In contrast to studies of the first women to use oral contraceptives, studies of the impact of more recent patterns of use (i.e., long-term exposures beginning early in life and before a full-term pregnancy) are in progress. Given that current low-dose oral contraceptive formulations will constitute the major proportion of all future exposures, and that studies to date have largely involved older, higher-dose formulations, studies of current (i.e., late 1980s and early 1990s) cohorts will be critical. Information about timing and duration of exposures will be particularly important and is likely to be equally—if not more—important than dosage in efforts to unravel early and late carcinogenic effects.

The committee considered efficient ways to obtain information about exposure, timing, and duration, and still ensure that any harmful effects will be detected in as short a time as possible. How long it will take to get the information is being dictated as much by the basic biology of breast cancer as by research design. The effort to untangle the relationship, if any, between oral contraceptives and breast cancer will be long and slow; to be successful, it must be comprehensive. Comprehensiveness requires that it be tightly linked to progress made in the overall understanding of the biology of the breast and the pathogenesis of the disease.

Data obtained from studies of different experimental mammals, although conflicting, suggest that some of the steroids used in oral contraceptives are capable of inducing tumors. A formal, four-step cancer risk assessment methodology (i.e., hazard identification, hazard characterization, exposure assessment, and risk characterization) has been used for more than 30 years by regulatory agencies. This risk assessment strategy extrapolates observed risk in animals to humans. The availability of human data from epidemiological studies allows for a desirable modification of the traditional approach.

The effect, if any, of oral contraceptives on breast cancer is perhaps the last substantial gap in knowledge of the side effects of the pill. The committee thus offers recommendations to address four policy issues related to diminishing that gap: (1) maintaining surveillance, (2) developing a broader array of contraceptives, (3) assessing knowledge for use in clinical practice, and (4) filling gaps in biological and epidemiological knowledge. The committee's recommendations are summarized in Table 1.

TABLE 1　Recommendations Made by the IOM Committee on the Relationship Between Oral Contraceptives and Breast Cancer

Maintaining surveillance

Recommendations

- Twenty to 40 years of epidemiological surveillance of appropriate cohorts to monitor risks and benefits of the long-term use of current and new formulations of the pill when used from an early age. This will assure the relative safety of all oral contraceptive formulations.
- Establish international, cooperative research in surveillance studies.
- Consideration of integration by the Food and Drug Administration of premarketing and postmarketing requirements to add greater emphasis on long-term safety.

Developing a broader array of contraceptives

Recommendation

- Research and development of a broader array of contraceptives, including more effective barrier and nonsteroidal methods.

Assessing knowledge for use in clinical practice

Recommendations

- The best available knowledge about oral contraceptives and breast cancer does not support any fundamental change in clinical practice with respect to use of oral contraceptives.
- Reassess this knowledge base at regular intervals and in light of new research results.
- Repeated NIH consensus conferences (beginning no later than three years hence) to regularly reassess guidelines for clinical practice.
- Improve dissemination of new and existing information about oral contraceptives and breast cancer among health care providers and women who use oral contraceptives.
- Provide women seeking contraception with adequate information and counseling relative to the current state of ambiguity with respect to the relationship between oral contraceptives and breast cancer.

Filling gaps in biological and epidemiological knowledge

Recommendations

- Multidisciplinary research initiatives to resolve the relationship between oral contraceptives and breast cancer.
- Implement a broad program of basic research in the biology of the breast.
- Use of classical epidemiologic approaches to analyze the relationship of oral contraceptives and breast cancer, including (i) a large, case-control study involving primarily women below the age of 45, and (ii) a study of postmenopausal women—who experience the bulk of breast cancer incidence.
- As biological markers become more generally available, they should be incorporated into epidemiological protocols.

MAINTAINING SURVEILLANCE

With oral contraceptives in widespread use, epidemiologists must maintain appropriate surveillance through the next 20 to 40 years to follow the effects of current and new formulations of the pill when used from an early age. They must also establish studies of risks and benefits to ensure the relative safety of new formulations. These future studies must (1) involve many thousands of cases and controls to permit statistically valid analyses of subgroups of users (e.g., individuals who used the pill prior to their first pregnancy), and (2) follow sufficient numbers of women for enough years to measure how long any possible effect persists after discontinuing oral contraceptive use. These are studies of daunting size and duration; nevertheless, they must be undertaken—and the necessary resources must be set aside to conduct them—to protect the health of American women.

The committee calls attention to the opportunity for international, cooperative research, owing to the complementarity of European and North American research data. There is enough variation in both exposure to oral contraceptives and opportunities for surveillance among the countries gathering data that a coordinated future research plan offers worldwide benefits. It is also important to note that some oral contraceptive formulations that are likely to become available in the United States over the next five years are already in use in a number of countries worldwide, including many European nations.

Further, the committee recommends that the Food and Drug Administration consider premarketing and postmarketing requirements as an integrated whole. There is a need to devise ways of spreading the investment already required by manufacturers, and ultimately paid for by users, in such a way as to maximize the information on safety that will result.

DEVELOPING A BROADER ARRAY OF CONTRACEPTIVES

The success and popularity of oral contraceptives as a means of avoiding conception are both a tribute to their efficacy and a reflection of the paucity of effective alternative means, particularly for young women. The committee underscores the urgent need for research and development of a broader array of contraceptives, including more effective barrier methods and nonsteroidal methods. It is not feasible to wait for resolution of the uncertainty about oral contraceptives as a potential risk factor for breast cancer before energizing research and development on alternative methods of contraception. In the face of uncertainty, those couples wishing to eschew oral contraceptives in favor of other methods of contraception must be served—and sooner, not later. Unless immediate steps are taken to develop a broader array of safe and effective contraceptives, the choice of contraceptives in the United States in the next century will not differ appreciably from the choice available today.

ASSESSING KNOWLEDGE FOR APPLICATION IN CLINICAL PRACTICE

The committee finds that, at the outset of the 1990s, the best available knowledge about oral contraceptives and breast cancer does not support any fundamental change in clinical practice with respect to use of the pill. This finding is subject to an important caveat: the knowledge base must be reassessed at regular intervals, in light of new research results (e.g., those forthcoming from the World Health Organization and the National Cancer Institute). The committee recommends that, three years hence, and at regular intervals thereafter, an NIH consensus conference reassess recommendations for oral contraceptive use based on reevaluation of the relationship between oral contraceptives and breast cancer. Two institutes in particular, the National Institute of Child Health and Human Development and the National Cancer Institute, would be appropriate lead institutes to judge when consensus conferences should be held. Current understanding of health benefits, as well as health risks, of oral contraceptives are described in detail in Appendix E and summarized in Chapter 4.

New research results should be periodically assessed for evidence of short- and long-term safety and carefully analyzed to provide clinicians with current information on the safest oral contraceptive use for younger and older women. There is also a need for continuous improvement of the dissemination of new and existing information about oral contraceptives and breast cancer among health care providers and women who use oral contraceptives. Multiple channels, through which providers and women can receive up-to-date information, must be opened and maintained. The committee emphasizes the obligation of all health care providers to offer adequate information to women seeking contraception and to counsel them regarding the current state of ambiguity with respect to the relationship between oral contraceptives and breast cancer. Only then can fully informed choices be made in clinical practice.

FILLING GAPS IN BIOLOGICAL AND EPIDEMIOLOGICAL KNOWLEDGE

The committee believes that a multidisciplinary research approach is necessary to resolve the relationship between oral contraceptives and breast cancer. Research on a broad front could well produce insights that would lead to some reduction in the incidence of breast cancer, in the same way that research throughout the past three decades has led to insights and changes of lifestyle that are today believed to be reducing the incidence of heart disease in America. With no single, "magic bullet" likely to prevent or cure breast cancer, the committee recommends a broad program of expanded studies on breast function and pathophysiology from the perspectives of endocrinology, biochemistry, molecular genetics, nutrition, cytology, and tissue culture.

Basic research in the biology of the breast is a priority. Research is especially needed on the transition from normal to abnormal growth, including, for example, research on the role of local growth factors and newly detected extracellular matrix proteins, estrogen metabolism, and oncogenes. As basic resources for this research, in vitro model systems that employ normal breast tissue are needed, in which the effects of oral contraceptive steroids can be directly examined.

Epidemiological research priorities include a large, case-control (retrospective) study with sufficient statistical power to resolve the assessment of small increases in relative risk of breast cancer. Such a study by the National Cancer Institute is in progress, involving primarily women below the age of 45. A study of postmenopausal women—who experience the bulk of breast cancer—is needed to elucidate the effects of (1) oral contraceptive use, and (2) oral contraceptive use followed by hormone replacement therapy. As oral contraceptive formulations and use patterns of the pill change, future case-control studies will be required. The launching of new cohort (prospective) studies is equal in priority to the conduct of case-control studies. There are no substitutes for these classical epidemiological approaches to resolving the relationship of oral contraceptives and breast cancer.

Biological markers, as they become more generally available, should be incorporated into epidemiological protocols. Consistent with a multidisciplinary approach to better understanding of the causes of breast cancer, there is a need for studies using biological markers within the context of epidemiological study designs, using innovative as well as traditional research tactics.

The expensive, complex program of studies necessary to reveal the relationship (if any) between oral contraceptives and breast cancer will inevitably draw on funding from several sources. The cost of such action must be weighed against the sobering costs of inaction: increased suffering and loss of life; the cost of treating breast cancer; and the cost of mammography screening programs, which lead to earlier detection but are not primary prevention. With oral contraceptives now being used by an estimated 10.7 million American women, any effect on breast cancer would be highly significant in terms of public health. Furthermore, any proven relationship or, what is equally important, any perceived relationship when one does not exist, would also have a marked effect on contraceptive practice in the United States.

1

Introduction and Overview

At least 50 million U.S. women have used oral contraceptives since they were introduced in 1960, and currently at least 10.7 million women depend on them for contraception (Mosher and Pratt, 1990). Eighty percent of all 35-year-old women use or have used them (Table 1-1; Dawson, 1990). The pattern of oral contraceptive use has changed over the years, however: less than 0.5 percent of women now aged 45-50 years used the pill prior to age 20, compared with 25 percent of women who are now 23 years old. Such shifts complicate analytic epidemiological studies of the short- and long-term effects of oral contraceptives. Younger women who have not yet started or have not yet completed their planned childbearing increasingly rely on oral contraceptives and other reversible methods of contraception, and women who do not plan further pregnancies rely more and more on irreversible sterilization procedures for themselves or their partners.

Breast cancer has become more common among American women through the twentieth century and now accounts for more of their new cases of cancer than are ascribed to cancer of any other organ (Figure 1-1). The rate among all women increased by 28 percent between 1974 and 1986 (Table 1-2), but the rates increased more in older than in younger women. Among women over age 50, the incidence of breast cancer has risen by approximately 1.4 percent a year since 1973 (Devesa et al., 1987); women age 50 and older now have 10 times the annual rate of women between the ages of 18 and 50 (Table

TABLE 1-1 Percentage of Women Who Have Ever Used Oral Contraceptives, by Birth Cohort and Marital Status, United States, 1987

Birth Cohort	Age at Interview (years)	All Women (percent)	Ever-married Women (percent)
1935-1939	48-52	46.9	47.9
1940-1944	43-47	67.9	70.7
1945-1949	38-42	80.6	81.9
1950-1954	33-37	80.6	82.7
1955-1959	28-32	79.4	82.9
1960-1964	23-27	78.2	85.4
1965-1969	18-22	49.5	80.4

SOURCE: Data from the 1987 National Health Interview Survey, adapted from D. A. Dawson, "Trends in Use of Oral Contraceptives—Data from the 1987 National Health Interview Survey," *Family Planning Perspectives* 22(1990):169-172.

1-3). Today, 1 in 9 women who live long enough develops the disease sometime in her life, and 1 in 18 can expect to die from it. Furthermore, approximately two-thirds of women over the age of 70 are reported to have abnormal cellular proliferation in their breast tissue (Kramer and Rush, 1973).

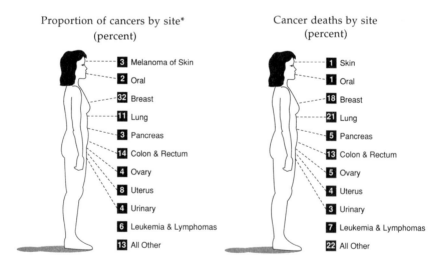

Proportion of cancers by site* (percent)

3	Melanoma of Skin
2	Oral
32	Breast
11	Lung
3	Pancreas
14	Colon & Rectum
4	Ovary
8	Uterus
4	Urinary
6	Leukemia & Lymphomas
13	All Other

Cancer deaths by site (percent)

1	Skin
1	Oral
18	Breast
21	Lung
5	Pancreas
13	Colon & Rectum
5	Ovary
4	Uterus
3	Urinary
7	Leukemia & Lymphomas
22	All Other

*Excluding nonmelanoma skin cancer and carcinoma in situ.

FIGURE 1-1 Estimates of cancer among American women, 1991. SOURCE: C. C. Boring, T. S. Squires, and T. Tong. "Cancer Statistics, 1991," *A Cancer Journal for Clinicians* 41(1991):19-51. Reproduced with permission of the American Cancer Society.

TABLE 1-2 Increases in Breast Cancer Incidence Rates Between 1974 and 1986

Age at Diagnosis	Percent Increase
25-44	15
45-54	6
55-64	20
65-74	40
75-84	30
Total	28

SOURCE: Emily White, Associate Member, Fred Hutchinson Cancer Research Center, Seattle, Washington, personal communication, 1990. Nine standard Surveillance, Epidemiology, and End Results (SEER) registries were used. Data were for females only, all races.

Thus, the introduction and dissemination of the use of oral contraceptives in the United States were superimposed on steadily rising breast cancer incidence rates (Devesa et al., 1987). In the United States, the years since the introduction of oral contraceptives have also been years in which hysterectomy and oophorectomy rates were increasing, and the prescription of replacement hormones (estrogens and progestins) for these and other postmenopausal women became widespread (Hemminki et al., 1988; Kennedy et al., 1985).

TABLE 1-3 Age-adjusted Breast Cancer Incidence Rates (per 100,000 women) for White Females; Surveillance, Epidemiology, and End Results Program

Year of Diagnosis	Age	
	Under 50	50 and Above
1973	29.1	252.1
1975	29.9	271.0
1977	28.8	258.4
1979	27.9	265.4
1981	28.8	280.3
1983	29.3	295.4
1985	32.0	326.7
Percent change	2.8	16.9
Average yearly change	0.2	1.4

SOURCE: Emily White, Associate Member, Fred Hutchinson Cancer Research Center, Seattle, Washington, personal communication, 1990 (data from National Cancer Institute, 1988).

The upward national trends in breast cancer incidence have continued and been consistently more marked in postmenopausal than in premenopausal women. The 1970s and 1980s were characterized by an acceleration of the increase in the U.S. postmenopausal breast cancer incidence rate, which has been more marked in women in their later 60s and 70s than in the earlier postmenopausal years. This is also the cohort of women who were too old ever to have taken oral contraceptives. The increase in annual numbers of cases, at least in postmenopausal women, is not completely explained by changes in age at first full-term pregnancy or wholly by increased rates of use of screening mammograms (The Cancer Letter, 1990; Marchant and Sutton, 1990; White et al., 1990). Nor, as yet, is any reason known for the apparently different experiences of younger and older postmenopausal women. Were older women exposed to an additional risk that bypassed younger cohorts? Has the effect of that additional risk yet to appear in younger cohorts? Were the younger cohorts exposed to that risk but protected against its effects by some new experience?

Against this background, the Institute of Medicine's Committee on the Relationship Between Oral Contraceptives and Breast Cancer assessed the role of oral contraceptives in breast cancer etiology. The committee met on three occasions through 1989 and 1990, convening an invitational conference in May 1990 to inform its deliberations. This report of the committee's efforts evaluates ways in which the etiology of breast cancer may relate to the use of oral contraceptives, identifies options for future research on several fronts, and lays out information for clinicians and women considering the use of the pill.

BIOLOGICAL PLAUSIBILITY OF A LINK
BETWEEN ORAL CONTRACEPTIVES AND BREAST CANCER

The etiology of breast cancer is unknown. Growth and differentiation of breast tissue are regulated by a large number of factors, including steroid hormones such as estradiol and progesterone. Therefore, it is biologically plausible that exogenously administered steroidal hormones such as those in the pill could have an effect on breast carcinogenesis. On purely theoretical grounds it is impossible to say whether this effect might be adverse or beneficial. Estrogen causes proliferation of breast tissue and would be expected to increase the risk of breast cancer by stimulating growth of stem and intermediate cells (Thomas, 1984). Progestin causes not only alveolar cell growth in the estrogen-primed breast but also differentiation. It is thus unclear whether the net effect would be to increase or decrease breast cancer risk (see Appendix A).

The finding of an oral contraceptive effect on breast cancer, however small and whether harmful or beneficial, could throw some general light on the pathogenesis of this devastating disease. Although a comprehensive evaluation of the possible etiologic mechanisms of breast cancer is beyond the scope of this report, clearly the uncertainty that currently exists about a possible interaction between this too-common cancer and the method of contraception used at one time or another by 80 percent of women in the United States must be resolved.

WHAT IS—AND IS NOT—KNOWN

Even though, over the past 30 years, oral contraceptives have become one of the most intensively studied drugs in history, the observational data collected to date are inadequate to answer the basic questions of whether oral contraceptives have an effect on the course of breast cancer and whether they make it more common or less common. About a dozen factors are at the core of what is—and is not—known.

The United States has one of the world's highest annual rates of breast cancer incidence, a rate that was already increasing steadily when oral contraceptives were introduced. Whether susceptible women had already fulfilled their carcinogenesis potential (see Appendix B) and could not react further to an added carcinogen, or whether it will simply take many more observations to measure a relatively small increment against an escalating high background rate, is hypothetical.

The age at which women have chosen to start using oral contraceptives has decreased (Table 1-4), and their pattern of use before the first pregnancy (Table 1-5) and to space pregnancies has changed. Younger women will need effective contraception for more than the average 5 years' use by older birth cohorts (Table 1-6). Studies to date have largely focused on patterns of use in years past and, although reassuring overall, do not address more recent patterns of use. In fact, the best existing information about oral contraceptives is for women now in their late 40s and early 50s—the first generation of oral contraceptive users in the 1960s—who used the pill to space their second and later pregnancies. Exposure to oral contraceptives around the time of menarche or menopause, or preceding the first full-term pregnancy, may have quite different influences.

Neither a positive nor negative association between overall breast cancer risk and oral contraceptive use has been found among the first generation of oral contraceptive users from the 1960s. These women lived in developed countries and used the pill for relatively short

TABLE 1-4 Cumulative Percentage of Women Who Have Ever Used Oral Contraceptives Prior to Selected Ages, by Birth Cohort, United States, 1987

Birth Cohort	Percent of Women Who Have Ever Used Oral Contraceptives Prior to Age:									
	15	18	20	25	30	35	40	45	50	55
1935-1939	0.0	0.1	0.3	8.9	28.9	39.9	45.0	46.5	46.9	46.9[a]
1940-1944	0.1	0.4	4.8	43.5	62.0	66.9	67.9	67.9	67.9[a]	
1945-1949	0.2	4.1	21.5	66.8	77.2	80.1	80.6	80.6[a]		
1950-1954	0.5	9.6	34.2	72.3	78.4	80.4	80.6[a]			
1955-1959	1.1	18.6	44.9	72.1	78.6	79.4[a]				
1960-1964	2.2	22.9	47.1	76.0	78.2[a]					
1965-1969	1.8	24.9	44.3	9.5[a]						

[a]This figure is a conservative estimate because not all women in the cohort have reached the age in question.

SOURCE: Data from the 1987 National Health Interview Survey, adapted from D. A.Dawson, "Trends in Use of Oral Contraceptives—Data from the 1987 National Health Interview Survey," *Family Planning Perspectives* 22(1990):169-172.

TABLE 1-5 Percent Distribution of Women Who Have Ever Used Oral Contraceptives, by Birth Cohort and by Timing of First Use, United States, 1987

Birth Cohort	Age at Interview (years)	Timing of Oral Conctaceptive Use		
		Before First Full-term Pregnancy (percent)	Same Age as Full-term Pregnancy (percent)	After First Full-term Pregnancy (percent)
1935-1939	48-52	11.9	3.4	84.7
1940-1944	43-47	31.7	7.5	60.8
1945-1949	38-42	53.2	12.2	34.6
1950-1954	33-37	67.3	11.7	21.0
1955-1959	28-32	72.0	9.9	18.1
1960-1964	23-27	75.8	10.6	13.6
1965-1969	18-22	77.3	12.8	9.9

SOURCE: Data from the 1987 National Health Interview Survey, adapted from D. A. Dawson, "Trends in Use of Oral Contraceptives—Data from the 1987 National Health Interview Survey," *Family Planning Perspectives* 22(1990):169-172.

TABLE 1-6 Women Who Have Ever Used Oral Contraceptives, by Birth Cohort, According to Average Months of Use, United States, 1987

Birth Cohort	Age at Interview (years)	Average Months of Use
1935-1939	48-52	51.3
1940-1944	43-47	60.8
1945-1949	38-42	60.6
1950-1954	33-37	56.2
1955-1959	28-32	52.7
1960-1964	23-27	38.0
1965-1969	18-22	24.3

SOURCE: Data from the 1987 National Health Interview Survey, adapted from D. A. Dawson, "Trends in Use of Oral Contraceptives—Data from the 1987 National Health Interview Survey," *Family Planning Perspectives* 22(1990):169-172.

periods of time—10 years being the longest exposure. Although there are no firm biological estimates of the longest latent periods between exposure and evidence of carcinogenesis, the existing 10 to 20 years of follow-up are probably sufficient to provide confidence in these results. An additional 5 to 10 years of follow-up of these first users would provide complete assurance of the safety of their use of oral contraceptives.

There is uncertainty about the relationship between oral contraceptive use and the relatively small number of breast cancers that arise in women under the age of 35. To date, studies have yielded inconsistent findings; some suggest an increased relative risk of breast cancer of as high as 1.6. Interpreting the positive findings in several recent case-control studies (see Appendixes A, B, and E) is difficult principally for two reasons. First, the positive subgroups keep changing. Second, the relative risk estimates are close to 1.0. Skegg (Appendix E, in this volume) warns that the relationship between oral contraceptives and breast cancer will not be clarified by chasing after "shifting goalposts" (i.e., positive subgroups). Rather, future studies should cover the full range of ages of women who have used the pill.

An important part of the information needed to resolve some of the uncertainties in the breast cancer/oral contraceptive question relates to duration and timing of exposure. Much more information is also needed about the effect on breast cancer incidence rates of short-term exposures at earlier ages (particularly before age 25 and/or before the first full-term pregnancy) on breast-cancer-incidence rates both before and after age 35. A further gap in knowledge is whether an increased risk detected before age 35 persists throughout the pre- and postmenopausal years. In line with these observations, more information is needed to learn whether oral contraceptive use increases risk in young women with diagnoses of benign breast disease even though breast cancer risk is increased only for women with specific histologic types of benign breast disease. The same information is needed about other breast cancer risk factors.

Although some information has been collected about the influence on breast cancer rates of relatively short-term exposures to oral contraceptives, whether long-term use beginning at any age increases pre-, peri-, or postmenopausal breast cancer risk has yet to be determined. And, the possibility has been raised that oral contraceptive use may increase breast cancer risk in relatively underdeveloped countries with low background breast cancer rates. This possibility also requires further inquiry.

If oral contraceptive use is associated with an increased risk of breast cancer at young ages, is this a promotional effect with a subsequent decrease in risk at older ages, or is this a cohort effect with an increased risk throughout the remainder of life? This question raises an issue of significant public health concern, given the current state of knowledge about oral contraceptives and breast cancer. Data from the Cancer and Steroid Hormone study support a promotional effect, but many other studies have not included women over the age of 35 or 45 and therefore do not have data to address the question. Furthermore, if changing patterns of oral contraceptive use (i.e., starting in the teenage years to delay a first pregnancy) or changing oral contraceptive composition (i.e., changing estrogen and progestin potencies) are related to increased risk at young ages, then it is only now—when the birth cohort who first experienced those use patterns enters its middle-aged years—that a cohort effect on breast cancer risk could be identified.

What are the effects on breast cancer risk of long-term oral contraceptive use followed by hormone replacement therapy? This question assumes particular importance because of the resurgence in popularity of hormone (i.e., estrogen or estrogen plus progestin) replacement therapy (HRT), and its recognized beneficial effects in prevention of osteoporosis and, for estrogen replacement therapy alone, prevention of cardiovascular disease. HRT is widely used: at least 15 percent of eligible women use it, or have used it, at some time; the percentage varies by geographic region within the United States. Furthermore, oral contraceptive users may be more likely than nonusers to use HRT subsequently. HRT itself has been evaluated in numerous studies for an effect on breast cancer risk. The findings have varied; some studies show small increased relative risk estimates (around 1.5 for long-term use), and others show no increase. However, there is only minimal information about the effects of HRT on the breast following prolonged use of oral contraceptives. The cohort of women with prolonged oral contraceptive use is just now entering the menopausal years when HRT is prescribed. This affords both the opportunity for and the necessity of studying breast cancer risk in relation to the use of oral contraceptives followed sequentially by HRT.

The preceding two questions are amenable to traditional epidemiological research designs—that is, case-control or cohort studies. An obvious strategy is a multicenter, case-control study of women aged 45-65. With this age group both types of hormonal products could be studied, and various details of HRT and oral contraceptive types and use patterns could be evaluated. Characteristics of the tumors—histology, stage, and receptor status—could be evaluated, provided the hypothesis, design, and power calculations allow for subgroup analyses. Furthermore, potential biases, such as source of controls and method of diagnosis, could be addressed in developmental phases and thus avoided in the main study.

Changes in oral contraceptive formulations stimulated a few of the existing epidemiological studies. It is now apparent that ethinyl estradiol and 19-nortestosterone derivatives are the most commonly used synthetic estrogen and progestin (see Appendix C). To date, no differences in possible associations with breast cancer have been observed between oral contraceptive formulations containing ethinyl estradiol and mestranol. Moreover, no 19-nortestosterone-derived progestin studied thus far has been shown to be more strongly associated with breast cancer than any other. Nevertheless, comprehensive studies of their specific effects are needed.

As a practical matter, physicians would like to be able to identify those women who could use the pill with absolute safety. Much more information is needed to help physicians identify women who are least likely to have their risk of breast cancer increased. Data are also necessary to determine oral contraceptive patterns of use that are least likely to increase risk and the influence of prior oral contraceptive use on the course of subsequent breast cancers.

Some of the questions noted above can be answered relatively quickly; others could take several decades of study in developed nations. A few of the questions may be best answered, and some can only be answered, in countries with relatively low background rates of breast cancer.

The epidemiology of breast cancer clearly suggests that hormone-related events during puberty, during fertile years around menopause, and after menopause can independently or synergistically influence breast cancer. Exposure information must therefore be collected throughout a majority of a woman's adult years, and the consequences of exposure must be monitored until the longest potential latent period has passed. Margins of 20 to 30 years must be used until there are better estimates of the shortest and longest intervals between exposures to carcinogens and promoters, and clinical diagnosis of breast cancer.

SEEKING ANSWERS

Premarketing drug testing is funded by the drug's developer or manufacturer. For safety's sake, all new drugs are tested on experimental animals prior to approval by the Food and Drug Administration (FDA) for first use in carefully controlled studies of human volunteers. Additional safety studies in animals are conducted, while human trials are ongoing, using many multiples of the human doses. Even so, safety is not necessarily ensured—for several reasons. The most important relates to the fact that different species of animals sometimes respond differently to the same drug, especially in the case of the reproductive system, for which variations among species are often widest. Human beings, for example, are the only primates whose breasts develop at puberty, instead of during the first pregnancy. Before manufacturers receive marketing approval from the FDA for a new drug or contraceptive, they must conduct trials of efficacy and safety on several hundred volunteers. Irrespective of cost, the scale and duration of such trials are insufficient to detect many rare, but potentially important, adverse or beneficial side effects. Although it is essential to gather as much relevant information as possible, every new drug widely used by the human species is an experiment that must be closely monitored. Nowhere is this fact more important than in the case of contraceptives, which are likely to be used at some time by a majority of adult women.

Once a drug is approved for marketing, there is generally no obligation on the part of manufacturers to conduct additional large-scale studies. However, medical research institutions, with private or federal funding, often carry out ad hoc investigations if pathology is suspected of being associated with use of the drug. In the case of oral contraceptives, a prudent alternative to waiting for the occurrence of unexpected disease is a well-planned cohort approach to detect all forms of unexpected side effects—and possible benefits, as well. Some such studies have been conducted in the United States and United Kingdom; investment in further cohort studies seems wise, particularly with new formulations of the pill becoming available and changes in use patterns.

Ecological data describing breast cancer incidence and mortality and oral contraceptive distribution and use are sparse, and they are likely to be of limited utility in countries with high rates of breast cancer. Whether they can be fully exploited worldwide will depend on the quality of national information systems. Chapter 2 explores this opportunity more fully. The chapter also discusses the need to plan a fresh cohort study as soon as a new oral contraceptive preparation is brought into general use, as well as the opportunity to capture essential new information that arises in countries that have relatively low background rates of breast cancer and that decide to introduce the pill as a generally available contraceptive.

The potential contributions of existing animal and in vitro human tissue models to questions of oral contraceptives and breast cancer have not been fully exploited, perhaps because they are mostly being used by investigators who are working within their own disciplines to answer other specific questions. Opportunities must be provided for interdisciplinary research that concentrates the expertise of investigators who use these models on efforts to get answers about oral contraceptives and breast cancer. These opportunities are discussed in Chapter 3. The existing evidence from animal models (see Appendix D) has been influential in continuing the effort to explore the possible influences of oral contraceptives on breast carcinogenesis.

Beside the rising rates of breast cancer incidence there is a virtual absence of definitive information about the pathological processes of breast carcinogenesis. Available experimental data from studies of different mammals are conflicting. However, the sum of the data suggests that some of the steroids used in oral contraceptives in certain dosage patterns are capable of inducing tumors in experimental animals. Both increased tumor incidence and decreased latency have been observed. Given the widespread use of these compounds, even a small increase in risk for lifetime cancer incidence would be expected to have a substantial effect on human populations using these hormones. This suggests that a careful, formalized risk assessment should be conducted and compared with the human epidemiological data. The assumptions for this risk assessment should be explicitly defined and delineated.

A formal, four-step cancer risk assessment methodology (comprising hazard identification, hazard characterization, exposure assessment, and risk characterization) has been used extensively over the past decade to protect the public health from known or suspected carcinogens (National Research Council, 1983, 1984). A modification of this approach that reflects the biology of the hormones found in oral contraceptives may be especially useful.

As mentioned earlier, breast cancer incidence rates increase steadily with age so that breast cancer is mainly a disease of the postmenopausal years (Table 1-7). A minority of breast cancer cases occur among women under the age of 45; therefore, most of the women who have had breast cancer since 1960 passed through their fertile years before oral contraceptives were widely used. Women now in their 40s, however, have used the pill more extensively and need answers to their questions about any possible interaction between the pill and breast cancer risk. In addition, if they use postmenopausal replacement hormones, questions about interaction with prior oral contraceptive use could become even more important.

When oral contraceptives were first approved for marketing by the FDA in 1960, they were known to be highly efficacious and thought by many not to have common, short-term, serious side effects. Little else was known about the more general effects of their use. With longer duration of use, an increasingly detailed picture of oral contraceptive risks and benefits is emerging (see Chapter 4). Today, practically the only important area to be resolved relates to breast cancer.

Overall, the pill has performed remarkably well as a relatively safe, effective, widely acceptable contraceptive (see Appendix E). Long-term follow-up has shown that oral contraceptive use can alter disease risk in pre- and perimenopausal women and that specific formulations modify these risks in different ways. The changes of greatest interest have been that certain types of cardiovascular disease have become more common and two reproductive cancers (i.e., ovarian and endometrial) have become less common. By developing different artificial hormones and reducing the amount of hormones in each tablet, some of the increased risk of cardiovascular disease observed in earlier, high-dose pills has been reduced without losing any of the cancer prevention benefits. Substantial gaps in data still exist, however. For example, although new progestins that are still making their way through the approval process in the United States have been widely used in Europe for a decade, there is no published body of epidemiological evidence on their influence on overall cardiovascular and cancer disease profiles. In addition, no postmenopausal women used oral contraceptives earlier in their reproductive lives for a period long enough to yield any information about systematic oral contraceptive influence on disease profiles. The lack of information on such influence applies not only to early but also to

TABLE 1-7   Breast Cancer Incidence
(per 100,000 women), United States, 1986

Age	Incidence Rate
20-24	1
25-29	7
30-34	30
35-39	65
40-44	131
45-49	186
50-54	217
55-59	263
60-64	331
65-69	402
70-74	424
75-79	450
80-84	443
85+	391

SOURCE: Nine standard Surveillance, Epidemiology, and End Results (SEER) registries. Females only, all races, by five-year age groups.

late postmenopausal years when coronary heart disease and breast
and ovarian cancers become more and more common.

Studies in the United States and around the world show that many
women—and some health care providers—are both misinformed and
unnecessarily pessimistic about the effects of the pill. For example,
fewer than a fifth of American women in 1987 (El Shafei et al., 1987)
knew that the pill protects against ovarian and uterine cancer; some
women considered oral contraceptive use to be more dangerous than
childbirth. (In fact, when the full range of proven side effects is
considered, childbirth is always more risky than using the pill [Fortney
et al., 1986].) In Chapter 4, the committee summarizes the best available information for pill users and health care providers.

Most of the relatively few unplanned pregnancies that do occur
during pill use are due to inconsistent or incorrect use, including
contemporaneous use of other drugs that compromise the effectiveness of oral contraceptives (Mattison, 1984). It is important to remember that users have not only fewer deliveries but fewer abor-
tions and ectopic pregnancies, each of which carries its own risk of
mortality and morbidity. In the short term, most women on the pill
have less menstrual loss, risk of anemia, and chance of acne, as well
as a reduction in premenstrual symptoms. Fewer pill users are hos-

pitalized for treatment of benign breast cysts. Users commonly complain that they are gaining weight on the pill, but this complaint has not been confirmed by the results of controlled trials. Some women do, however, suffer an increase in blood pressure, which can become a reason to stop pill use.

Initial oral contraceptive use can be associated with nausea and breast tenderness. Serious side effects include an increased risk of heart attack and stroke, with their associated mortality and morbidity, and of clotting in the deep veins of the leg which, in the rare event that a large clot dislodges, can also lead to death. The risk of adverse cardiovascular effects begins more or less as soon as the user takes her first pill and is thought to disappear shortly after she takes her last tablet. The cardiovascular risk of using the pill rises steeply in the 40s and interacts in an especially powerful way with cigarette smoking. Even for women over 40, the benefits of the pill often continue to outweigh the risks, as long as they are nonsmokers. Smokers of this age—if they cannot stop smoking—should use an alternative method of contraception. Pill users have more gall bladder disease than nonusers of the same age, most probably because use advances a disease that would otherwise have appeared somewhat later in the life of the same woman. Oral contraceptives are associated with a marked increase in the relative risk of benign and malignant liver tumors, but these tumors are so exceedingly rare among U.S. women that a pill user's absolute risk of getting one remains low.

It is always easier to record a case of disease than the fact that a disease did not occur. Twenty years' work was required to demonstrate that oral contraceptives protect against developing ovarian and endometrial cancer years after oral contraceptive use, whereas it took less than 10 years to demonstrate some of the pill's adverse effects on the cardiovascular system. Fortunately, although cardiovascular risks arise when the pill is first used, they also fall soon after its use is stopped; on the other hand, the cancer protection benefits take some years of use to build up and, in contrast to the cardiovascular effects, persist for many years after taking the last pill. Seven years' use of oral contraceptives reduces the risk of ovarian cancer by 60 to 80 percent during the next 10 years. Only 4 percent of cancers among American women are ovarian, but the disease has already spread to other organs in 60 percent of women at the time of diagnosis. In addition to cancer protection, pill users also have less pelvic inflammatory disease, although this effect is probably a consequence of changes in the cervical mucus, which begin and end with oral contraceptive use.

In addition to the unresolved questions concerning the pill and breast cancer, there is also a lack of scientific agreement about the possible influence of oral contraceptives on cervical cancer. The pill could have an effect on cervical changes, although a growing understanding of the etiology of cervical cancer points to involvement of the human papilloma virus (HPV). Of course, the involvements of HPV and oral contraceptives are not mutually exclusive. The overall incidence of death owing to invasive cervical cancer is decreasing, and it is less threatening because early detection can lead to its complete cure. Scientists disagree about the influence of the pill because the higher prevalence of cervical cancer reported among pill users in several studies may be due to confounding factors, in particular, the possibility that oral contraceptive users may have more sexual partners than nonusers and that they may have cervical smears taken more frequently.

Research into the causes and mechanisms of breast cancer, particularly in relation to the large increase in the incidence of the disease, has been conducted in an ad hoc fashion without any long-term investment in a coherent, national multidisciplinary research program. Further, the development of research resources and technologies needs to support such a program and carry it to the cutting edge of 1990s' state of the art. Chapter 5 addresses the critical question of resources for future research.

It is interesting to note that the relationship of oral contraceptives and breast cancer is not the only area of epidemiological investigation that has proved difficult and occasionally yielded contradictory results. In 1970, a large multicenter trial (MacMahon et al., 1970) was unable to demonstrate any relationship between breastfeeding and breast cancer. Further work was not conducted until the 1980s, when two studies from different parts of the world demonstrated a strongly protective, dose-dependent effect of lactation on the subsequent risk of breast cancer (McTiernan and Thomas, 1986; Yuan et al., 1988). Not long afterward, another group (London et al., 1990) was unable to confirm these results. Clearly, breastfeeding is a variable that needs to receive greater priority in all studies, including those that involve the pill and breast cancer.

Oral contraceptives have proved popular not only in America but in diverse cultures ranging from China to Indonesia to Tunisia to Colombia, and their use is likely to continue to grow rapidly in the coming decade. Globally, one woman a minute dies from pregnancy, childbirth, or abortion, and there is no doubt that oral contraceptives have saved and will continue to save a great many lives. Research continues, albeit at a low level, into new methods of contraception, and additional contraceptive choices would be welcome (NRC/IOM,

1990). At the same time, even though there remain key unanswered questions about oral contraceptives and breast cancer, it must be noted that any new methods, such as progestin-only subdermal implants, will require a whole new generation of investigations—and investigators—to illuminate the same set of unknowns that surrounded the introduction of the first oral contraceptives 30 years ago. It is imperative to fill in what is possibly the last substantial gap in knowledge of oral contraceptive side effects—namely, the effect, if any, on breast cancer. More than 80 percent of American women now in their 20s and 30s who have ever had intercourse have used the pill at some time or other in their fertile lives. Scientific study of the pill and of breast cancer, separately and combined, are therefore topics of immense and urgent importance to rapidly increasing numbers of American women.

2

Epidemiology: Information Needs and Data Gaps

With limited observational data about the influence of widespread use of oral contraceptives on breast cancer incidence and mortality, almost the entire body of scientific information about the influence of oral contraceptive use on the relative risk of breast cancer can be found in about a dozen research reports. These studies were all carried out in developed nations and are either population-based, hospital-based case-control, or cohort designs (see Appendix B). There are also a few case-control studies from developing nations. The present system of small, ad hoc studies is unsatisfactory, and there is a need for more, long-term, systematically coordinated epidemiological studies with sufficient statistical power.

EPIDEMIOLOGICAL RESEARCH

Epidemiology is the scientific study of the distribution and determinants of disease in populations. As a science of public health it employs research methods derived from many other fields such as survey research, biology, toxicology, and statistics. It attempts to integrate the available data so as to answer important questions about health. Although the experimental method can sometimes be employed, observational methods are often the only possible research strategy, especially when adverse effects are under investigation. The principal methods used by epidemiologists are the case-control (retrospective) method, the cohort (prospective) method, and ecological

25

methods in which trends of exposure and disease in populations are correlated. The application of these methods in efforts to shed light on the question of the possible association of oral contraceptives and breast cancer is discussed in the following sections.

Case-Control Method

The case-control method compares the previous use of birth control methods by women with breast cancer and a comparison group. This method is the most efficient in terms of both time and cost, but it is limited in the number of adverse or beneficial effects it can measure. One of its greatest disadvantages is the poor documentation of prescriptions for oral contraceptives and the likelihood that women who do not use the pill have other characteristics or conditions that make them inappropriate for purposes of comparison.

The number of cases of breast cancer and of controls needed to obtain statistically sound results depends on the prevalence of exposure to oral contraceptives and not on the rarity of the disease. It is not surprising, therefore, that much of what is known about oral contraceptives comes from case-control studies. Given the disadvantages of the case-control method, it is also not surprising that there is little or no scientific information about the results of long-term exposure.

Case-control studies have been proven reliable guides when the detected relative risks are moderate or large, but a problem emerges when the relative risks are small or marginal. In these cases, the possibility that bias of some sort may have led to the finding of increased risk is a more tenable alternative hypothesis than when the relative risks are large.

In the matter of the relation of oral contraceptives to breast cancer the relative risks have been either modest or small, and they have not been found consistently. This situation has created uncertainty about the meaning of some of the "positive" studies. One approach to sorting out inconsistent replications of small risk measurements is to initiate a large, case-control study with sufficient statistical power to resolve the matter. The National Cancer Institute's new, large (2,000 cases), case-control study is just such an effort (Brinton, 1990). In addition to this large study, it is highly likely that future case-control studies will be required as oral contraceptive formulations and use patterns change.

Seven strategies are likely to improve future case-control studies:

• standardized history-taking using pictures of the oral contraceptive formulations so that analysis by formulation is possible;

- attempts to validate complete contraceptive history;
- information-gathering about histopathology of tumors, if possible;
- use of biological markers (when and if these become available) and other laboratory methods to help categorize risk group;
- studies in populations that use oral contraceptives but that have much lower incidence rates of breast cancer than most Western countries;
- regular studies that employ comparable methods of information-gathering (because of the problem of changing formulations, changing use patterns, and long length of time from tumor induction or promotion to tumor diagnosis); and
- use of information about screening and earlier diagnosis to correct for possible "early diagnostic bias" arising from selective screening exams (and more sensitive screening devices) applied to oral contraceptive users now that the possible link between oral contraceptives and cancer has been widely publicized.

Cohort Studies

There have been few cohort investigations of the relationship between oral contraceptives and breast cancer because of the large number of women who must be followed for so many years. Even when such longitudinal studies are possible, their statistical power is unlikely to be large; thus, the hope of identifying small risks is quite low. Nevertheless, the cohort design has the advantages of allowing better evaluation of the role of bias and easier validation of exposure histories. The use of telephone and mail to follow up large cohorts has been shown to be practical in the Nurses Health Studies I and II in Boston (Romieu et al., 1990), the Family Planning Study at Oxford (McPherson, 1990; Vessey, 1990), and the cohort assembled by the Royal College of General Practitioners (Kay, 1990).

Other opportunities for cohort-type research, either prospective or "historical," arise through prepaid health plans and data linkage systems that include information about drug prescription and cancer incidence. Examples include the Saskatchewan data base in Canada, the population-based data systems of the Uppsala region of Sweden, and large, closed health maintenance organizations (HMOs) in the United States (e.g., Kaiser Permanente in California; Group Health Cooperative of Puget Sound).

A special category of cohort studies is postmarketing surveillance following the introduction of new contraceptives. This surveillance should be required for oral contraceptives that contain new hormonal constituents or for those with significant alterations in the existing formulations. The plan for such an effort must be based on sound epidemiological principles and would bear little resemblance to current postmarketing surveillance, which often amounts to little more than sporadic reporting of adverse drug reactions or company-conducted marketing studies.

Comparison Groups

Case-control and cohort studies share a significant methodological problem: uncertainty as to how to choose the comparison group. The usual strategy is to compare disease occurrence among the exposed population relative to the nonexposed population. With oral contraceptives, the issue is complicated because the majority of women in this country have used the pill; those who have not may not be representative of the general population of women (for additional discussion, see Appendix A). Furthermore, the ways in which nonusers are unrepresentative will vary, so that the direction of the bias is not easily known in advance. Nonusers may include women of both high and low social class, health-conscious women, women with medically diagnosed illnesses, women who abstain from sexual activity, infertile women, and women with family histories of cancer and cardiovascular disease. These factors and others, such as frequency of mammography, may relate to risk of breast cancer and rates of detection; consequently, their variable distribution in non-oral-contraceptive-using women could seriously distort the estimates of effect—that is, breast cancer risk estimates—if nonusers are the comparison group.

Short-term users of oral contraceptives may also be a poor choice as a comparison group because they probably include a large segment of women who for medical reasons or perceived symptoms discontinued oral contraceptive use soon after starting it. In sum, there is not an obvious solution to the problem of choice of a comparison group in case-control and cohort studies.

Ecological Studies

Ecological studies correlating trends in breast cancer incidence rates with trends in oral contraceptive use have not been informative in the past and are unlikely to be so in the future, except possibly in developing countries where the underlying breast cancer rates are low. (On the other hand, in developing countries the cancer information systems are unreliable, so useful data generally will be lacking.)

The reason for the probable lack of utility of this method is that, in developed countries, it is unlikely that any influence on breast cancer rates would be large and clear enough to be distinguished from other influences. This indistinguishability is in contrast to the situation of pulmonary embolism in young women, for which the effect of oral contraceptives was detected. In that instance, the risk was fairly large, immediate, and led to sudden death, and the underlying rates were low. Cancer of the endometrium was another such case: there, the widespread use of replacement hormones was age-specific and increased rapidly in a short time.

Special Studies

Women Exposed to Hormones Other than Oral Contraceptives

Opportunities exist to study women who have been heavily exposed to hormones. Some are endogenously exposed (e.g., women with polycystic ovaries), and others are exogenously exposed (e.g., women with Turner's syndrome who have been treated with steroid hormones, girls given estrogens to stop their long bone growth, or women given diethylstilbestrol (DES) during pregnancy). In the case of DES, both the exposed women and their progeny, male and female, can be followed. Such studies can employ traditional epidemiological designs, comparing exposed subjects with nonexposed subjects for subsequent risk of breast cancer. Controls can be internal (e.g., pregnant women who were not exposed to DES from the same time period and hospital as those who were exposed), or external, which is often a statistical estimate based on the breast cancer experience of a large population. In these heavily exposed populations, investigators can evaluate the direct effects of particular hormones on breast cancer risk, but the issue of inferring that these results pertain to oral contraceptive use remains.

Women Genetically Susceptible to Breast Cancer

Are there differences in susceptibility among oral contraceptive users who do and do not get breast cancer? Or, alternatively, among women with a high risk for breast cancer, does oral contraceptive use further increase that risk?

These questions arise from an inference that seems logical, given the existing data. Breast cancer occurrence before the age of 40 or even 45 is a rare event. Only 15 percent of all breast cancers occur before age 45. Let us suppose that there is a small increase in the frequency of these cancers in association with long-term oral contraceptive use, as some studies have suggested. This small increase is occurring in conjunction with a high use prevalence of oral contraceptives, 50 to 70 percent of all women currently less than age 45, the exact percentage depending on the exact age. Given a small increase in the occurrence of a rare event resulting from an extremely common exposure, what is the likelihood that the excess events are randomly distributed in the exposed population versus the likelihood that only a small segment of the exposed population is at high risk of incurring breast cancer at an early age? Irrespective of oral contraceptive use, the occurrence of breast cancer at young ages is more likely to have a strong family history of the disease, to be present in breast cancer families (i.e., pedigrees), and to be associated with known genetic syndromes (e.g., ataxia telangiectasia—a DNA repair deficiency). Thus, genetic susceptibility factors are thought to be much more strongly associated with early-onset than with late-onset disease. The possibility of an interaction between oral contraceptive use and other biological phenomena, which are most likely genetically determined, necessitates some additional types of studies.

To characterize genetic susceptibility and study its interaction with oral contraceptives will require specialized populations and innovative methodologies. For example, one might identify patients and pedigrees with genetic syndromes that are known to confer a high risk of breast cancer, such as a DNA repair deficiency, or heterozygotes and ask: Does oral contraceptive use increase this risk further? What is the breast cancer risk in oral contraceptive users versus nonusers in families with known DNA repair deficiencies (e.g., ataxia telangiectasia families)? To the extent that assays are available to detect molecular alterations that increase breast cancer risk or closely linked molecular markers, four groups of women could be formed and followed for breast cancer occurrence: women with and without the marker, divided into oral contraceptive users and nonusers. If the marker assays are complex, limiting the number that can be performed, studies of oral contraceptive users only would be informative.

It is important to recognize that the current capability of molecular technology may not be adequate to characterize susceptibility (see Chapter 3). In that event, other options are needed for characterizing susceptible women. High-risk phenotypes may be characterized using more traditional methods. As an example, the ongoing National Cancer Institute study of breast cancer and oral contraceptives in women under 45 years of age could serve as a source of subjects. One could identify very young cases and controls with one or two first-degree relatives with breast cancer diagnosed at a young age (specific criteria to be defined). If oral contraceptives interact with susceptibility, the increased risk should be observable in this restricted population.

An alternative strategy derived from a large case-control study might use the same criteria for identifying susceptible cases but use phenotypically normal sisters as controls. Ideally, a genetic analysis (e.g., restriction fragment length polymorphism) of both case and control subjects would be performed to detect specific molecular alterations. In addition, or alternatively, linkage analyses could be done.

Molecular markers for mutational effects (i.e., oncogene activation), loss of heterozygosity, or polymorphisms (i.e., alleles) can be sought, given the availability of appropriate assays. One such study of traditional case-control design is currently in progress, funded by the National Cancer Institute. Rare alleles of Ha-*ras* are being sought as susceptibility markers with oral contraceptives being considered as effect modifiers (Garrett and Hulka, personal communication).

One innovative strategy (Swift et al., 1990) tests hypothesized associations between a candidate allele, for which there is a specific laboratory test, and a common chronic disease, such as breast cancer. Families in which this allele is segregating are identified through index individuals who are heterozygous or homozygous for the allele. One relative with the disease of interest (e.g., breast cancer) must be available for each index case. The proportion of heterozygotes observed in the diseased sample is compared with the expected proportion, based on each diseased relative's null probability. The advantage of this strategy over a more traditional case-control approach is the reduction in sample size required to test the hypothesis of a specific allele rendering susceptibility to breast cancer.

To enhance the capability of molecular epidemiological research, the molecular characterization of breast cancer in oral contraceptive users and nonusers is needed. If polymerase chain reaction can be used and restriction fragment length polymorphisms can be studied using formalin-fixed tissues, existing repositories of tumor samples (i.e., clinical pathology laboratories) could provide expanded opportunities for these studies (Frye et al., 1989; Resnick et al., 1990). Whatever study design and epidemiological strategy are used, every attempt should be made to observe the influence of oral contraceptive use on specific types of malignant breast tumors, using the best generally available technology.

Estrogen Metabolism

Estrogen metabolism may figure prominently in future epidemiological research. Fishman and colleagues (1984) have proposed that breast cancer patients, in comparison with normal controls, have higher levels of the 16α-hydroxyestrone metabolite and lower levels of the 2-OH metabolite of estrone. These results need to be replicated in larger studies and the effect of oral contraceptive use on the levels of these metabolites explored. An alternative to the existing radiometric assay is required to evaluate these estrogen metabolites in epidemiological studies using blood or urine samples as the biological medium. Furthermore, it has been stated that the 16α-hydroxyestrone metabolite can form permanent, covalent adducts with the E2 receptor, turning on the receptor indefinitely. This metabolite is also said to form adducts with albumin and hemoglobin. Because a variety of assays for adduct formation are available, additional clarification of these issues would be useful for future epidemiological research. For example, levels of estrogen-metabolite adduct formation in breast tumor and normal tissue from oral contraceptive-using and non-oral contraceptive-using patients could provide suggestive information on the carcinogenic potential of these metabolites.

Progestins

Further studies are needed of the biological effects of the progestin component of oral contraceptives and its interaction with the estrogen component. This effort should be tackled from an interdisciplinary perspective using more combined, in vivo/in vitro studies of endogenous and exogenous hormone effects on human breast epithelial cells. Through use of the thymidine labeling index (TLI), epithelial proliferation of normal breast lobules has been shown to change over the menstrual cycle (Anderson et al., 1990). Proliferation is increased in the second half of the monthly cycle—when progesterone levels are elevated. Furthermore, breast epithelium from young women was shown to be more responsive than that of older women. Nulliparous oral contraceptive users had a significantly greater increase in TLI than their parous counterparts during the last week of their "cycle" (i.e., the equivalent of the late secretory phase of a normal cycle). High-dose estrogen oral contraceptives may cause more proliferation than oral contraceptives with lower estrogen dosages, but there were no significant differences among progestins. This avenue of investigation needs to be extended more broadly in the future to further document the differences between parous and nulliparous women, and to include more data on a variety of oral contraceptive formulations. Such studies should be designed to gather additional data such as blood and tissue levels of endogenous or exogenous hormones (at the time of diagnostic biopsy) that are critical to the interpretation of these findings.

Changing Oral Contraceptive Formulations

In recent reviews of the existing case-control and cohort studies of the influence of oral contraceptives on the relative risk of breast cancer, a great deal of concern has been expressed about the constraints placed on investigators by changes in oral contraceptive formulations and inconsistent methods of recording ages and patterns of use. (The evolving formulations of oral contraceptives are described in Appendix C.) These concerns have centered on oral contraceptives themselves; investigators now need to ask whether subsequent hormone replacement therapy with differing duration of use and differing formulations (in the presence or absence of oophorectomy) modifies the long-term oral contraceptive effects. Attention must be paid to the sample sizes needed in cohort or case-control studies to measure a specified effect against differential background trends and sequential confounding or modifying exposures.

SUMMARY AND CONCLUSIONS

There is a continuing need for well-designed observational epidemiological studies of the relationship of oral contraceptives to breast cancer. As new formulations are introduced, continued postmarketing surveillance must be carried out; this surveillance is particularly important because of emerging patterns of long-term use and increasing use of hormone replacement therapy during menopause. It is possible that newer techniques derived from the explosion of knowledge in molecular biology may become useful in epidemiological investigations.

The lack of precision surrounding small risks can be overcome by large-scale studies. The possibly long latency periods can be addressed by following cohorts for substantial periods of time and periodically repeating case-control studies. In addition, new cohort studies must be initiated to gather information about new formulations and use patterns.

The problem of the relationship between oral contraceptives and breast cancer illustrates both the complexity of biological interrelationships and the difficulties inherent in monitoring long-term exposures of human populations in a modern, mobile society that can quickly change its contraceptive practices and patterns of use of exogenous hormones.

Current knowledge of the putative relationship comes from complementary studies of exposures in Northern Europe, the United States, and developing countries. Future studies should continue to capitalize on these complementary opportunities (e.g., the advanced use of new formulations in Europe and variations in background breast cancer incidence rates). The potential to maximize future knowledge by planned coordination of international research should be explored most immediately in the United Kingdom and the United States.

The cost of long-term prospective studies is driven by the number of people who must be tracked and the number of years tracking must be maintained. For the purposes of these studies, breast cancer is relatively uncommon; thus, large numbers of women must be followed—making studies of breast-cancer incidence unavoidably expensive. Research costs can be contained by careful selection of study populations and sources of information about outcome measures. National, regional, or institutionally defined populations with linked record systems offer the best opportunity for relatively low-cost collection of information about exposure and, in some cases, outcomes. Population-based cancer registries such as the Surveillance, Epidemiology, and End Results (SEER) program provide an important resource for identification of cancer cases. It may be more cost-efficient to provide support to maintain the integrity of these sources of subjects, information, and events than to establish entirely new, dedicated recruitment, collection, and follow-up systems. In the United States, particular consideration should be given to the populations of large, comprehensive, closed health maintenance organizations within SEER collection areas.

3

Biology: Information Needs
and Data Gaps

Mammary tissue undergoes a complex process of development during embryonic life. Studies in the mouse and rat have indicated that normal development and differentiation depend on interactions among three cell types (epithelial, myoepithelial, and stromal) and hormones reaching these cells through the bloodstream.

Human mammary tissue undergoes a major developmental change around puberty, when ovarian steroid hormone levels increase and menstrual cycles begin. The development process occurs in response to, and is critically dependent on, the complex interaction of a large number of systemic hormones as well as local regulatory factors. Changing levels of ovarian steroids and anterior pituitary hormones during the menstrual cycle alter all hormone target tissues in the body. Breast tissue shows differences in mitotic index, estrogen and progesterone receptor levels, and various intracellular metabolites during the follicular and luteal phases that follow the cyclic changes in estrogen and progesterone levels. Pregnancy, with its increasing steroid and lactogenic hormone secretion from the placenta, leads to increased mammary ductile development. After pregnancy, the hormonal milieu of lactation leads to synthesis and secretion of milk from epithelial cells. Thus, throughout ontogeny, mammary cells are subject to changing concentrations of pituitary, ovarian, and placental hormones that interact to modulate cellular differentiation and function. The synthetic hormones contained in oral contraceptives simulate the natural steroid hormones secreted by the ovaries and placenta.

This chapter—which raises more questions than it answers—defines an agenda for the basic research in biology that will be required to fully understand the relationship between oral contraceptives and breast cancer.

SIGNAL COMPLEXITY IN BREAST REGULATION

The complexity of regulation of breast physiology may exceed that of any other hormonal target tissue (Table 3-1). The effects of both classical hormones and a variety of growth hormones on growth and function of breast tissue and cells have been extensively studied. Classical hormones cause growth, differentiation, and milk synthesis and secretion, and include hormones from the anterior pituitary (prolactin, growth hormone), ovary (estrogen, progesterone, relaxin), placenta (placental lactogen[s], growth hormone), adrenal cortex, thyroid, and pancreas. These hormones may act directly on specific pathways of metabolism and cell division within the breast, or they may work indirectly through locally secreted growth factors (see below), which, in turn, regulate cell function. Additionally, the hormones and growth factors may interact with and modify each other's effects, changing secretion rates and actions (e.g., estrogens increasing prolactin secretion and tissue receptors for progesterone).

Growth hormones or factors are peptides secreted by most, if not all, cells. They are essential for growth and differentiation of many tissues. Unlike the classical hormones, these substances were discovered only after it was noted that many cells in culture in chemically defined media were incapable of growth, cell division, or differentiation without the addition of serum from animals. Growth factors can act as local growth regulators and can inhibit or stimulate mitogenesis of epithelial or stromal cells; they can also stimulate angiogenesis and influence cell transformation and immortalization.

In culture, normal or malignant breast tissue can secrete transforming growth factors (TGF-α) or (TGF-β), epidermal growth factor (EGF), insulin-like growth factors (IGF-I and IGF-II), platelet-derived growth factor (PDGF), and fibroblast growth factor (FGF) under various conditions. These factors can act as paracrine and autocrine growth regulators. TGF-β has been shown to act normally as an inhibitor of mammary gland growth, whereas EGF acts as a stimulator of mammary growth (Lippman and Dickson, 1989).

Recent work suggests that hormones (e.g., estrogen) may in some cases act by changing growth factor secretion locally, and perhaps by changing receptors for these factors as well. The observation that estrogen receptors in stromal tissue may be responsible for differen-

TABLE 3-1 Growth Factors and Hormones Potentially Involved in Breast Development and Differentiation

Transforming growth factor α	Growth hormone
Transforming growth factor β	Prolactin and other lactogens
Insulin-like growth factor I	Relaxin
Insulin-like growth factor II	Somatostatin
Fibroblast growth factor	Thyroid hormone
Rochefort's 52-K protein	Gonadotropins
Epidermal growth factor	Estrogens
Platelet-derived growth factor	Progestins
Insulin	Corticoids

SOURCE: Adapted from K. S. McCarty, Jr., "Proliferative Stimuli in the Normal Breast: Estrogen or Progestins?," *Human Pathology* 20(1989):1137-1138.

tiation of epithelial tissue by means of some paracrine influence speaks to the complexity of the regulation of breast tissue.

Another new paradigm is the importance of extracellular matrix (ECM) proteins in influencing cell-cell interactions and in defining "tissues." The extracellular matrix is the conglomeration of substances on which cells sit and which ties them together as a "tissue." The proteins of the matrix are secreted locally and provide yet another means of cell-cell communication. The production of these proteins is regulated by the cells that produce them; in turn, the proteins regulate the function and differentiation of the cells that constitute the tissue. In the absence of extracellular matrix proteins, many cells, including cells of mammary tissue, do not show normal morphology and organization. Extracellular matrix proteins include collagens, laminin, fibronectin, glycosaminoglycans, and probably many others. They influence not only mammary tissue morphology in culture but also function, increasing greatly the synthesis of proteins responsible for milk secretion, including a primary constituent of milk, casein. In a number of tissues, including breast epithelium, it has been observed in vitro that normal epithelial function, such as secretion or differentiation, does not take place unless a normal extracellular matrix is present.

Many hormone effects on target cells are mediated by actions of ECM protein secretions, or by secretion of growth factors locally. Normal breast morphology and function can only be understood by factoring these local signals into our total understanding. Perhaps the apparent heterogeneity of breast cancer etiology (i.e., the wide range of cell types and receptors involved) may be understandable in terms of these local signals.

RESEARCH ISSUES

Until recently, the question before this committee as to whether oral contraceptives influence the risk of breast cancer could be addressed only by human epidemiological and animal studies. Human epidemiological studies (see Chapter 2) are and will remain the central source of information concerning the link, if any, between oral contraceptives and breast cancer. Rapid advances in molecular endocrinology and in the biochemistry and biology of growth factors and steroid and peptide hormones now permit scientists to gain some insight into the biological links between breast neoplasia and oral contraceptives. This knowledge should provide a rationale and hence support for epidemiological observations, and also allow the construction of biological hypotheses that can then be subjected to testing through epidemiological studies.

Numerous positive animal studies have focused attention on the estrogens in oral contraceptives as possibly being involved in breast cancer. Although much in vivo animal evidence shows that estrogens have a causative or permissive effect on mammary tumors, there is no comparable information for humans. Yet indirect evidence, mostly in the form of epidemiological data, exists for a relationship between human breast cancer and ovarian steroids, particularly estrogens. The disease is far more prevalent in women than in men, with a ratio of 100 to 1. Ovariectomy in early reproductive years decreases risk. Moreover, the relationship between the estrogen receptor in the tumor and its response to hormonal treatment implies a hormonal link to breast cancer.

The putative association between the estrogens in oral contraceptives and human breast cancer could be the result of quantitative, temporal, or qualitative factors. The quantitative relationship appears to be the least likely because the effect of the oral contraceptives is to depress the endogenous ovarian production of the natural hormone estradiol. The low-dose estrogen pill (see Appendix C) contains less estrogen than the average follicular-stage daily production rate of estradiol (about 80 micrograms per day [μg/day] during the early follicular phase) and much less than the preovulatory secretion in the human and the secondary luteal rise of the hormone, both of which are extinguished by the exogenous hormone. Pharmacokinetic studies with oral contraceptives containing 30-35 μg of estrogen suggest that the average serum concentration of ethinyl estradiol is similar to midfollicular-phase levels of estradiol and less than peak preovulatory levels. Therefore, it might be inferred that the net effect of low-dose and triphasic oral contraceptives is to decrease estrogen "load." However, there is marked inter- and intraindividual variability in pharmacokinetic profiles following oral contraceptive ingestion.

Oral contraceptives disrupt the cyclical nature of estrogen secretion of a normal ovulatory cycle and replace it with a relatively constant level over 20 days. Whether this temporal change might be responsible for differential cellular changes in breast cells is not known. However, pregnancy, with its noncyclical, high estrogen levels for as long as six to nine months, has not been associated with increased risk—but rather with decreased risk. Ovariectomy, which results in a constant, low background level of estrogens derived from peripheral aromatization, is also associated with decreased risk for breast cancer.

The qualitative aspects of a possible link between the synthetic estrogen in oral contraceptives and breast cancer derive from structural differences between the synthetic and the endogenous hormone. Although present knowledge indicates that the interaction of 17α-ethinyl estradiol and its prodrug, mestranol, with the estrogen receptor parallels that of estradiol in the qualitative sense, there are major differences in the metabolism of the natural hormone and ethinyl estradiol that may impinge on their biological properties. The metabolism of estradiol in the human is largely oxidative in nature. Estradiol is oxidized to estrone in a reversible reaction, but the equilibrium is greatly in favor of estrone. This metabolic transformation cannot occur in the 17α-ethinyl estrogens. Estrone is then irreversibly transformed by two largely competitive hydroxylations. Hydroxylation at C-2 leads to catechol estrogens which are ineffective as estrogen agonists, whereas hydroxylation at 16α leads to 16α-hydroxyestrone and estriol, which are potent estrogens with some unusual biological features. The 17α-ethinyl estrogens in oral contraceptives are metabolized primarily by the 2-hydroxylative route with minimal 16α hydroxylation.

The difference in metabolic pathways between the natural and the synthetic estrogens could have important biological consequences and may be relevant to the occurrence of breast cancer. Some evidence suggests that a product of 16α hydroxylation interacts in a covalent fashion with the estrogen receptor, which might lead to genomic consequences different from those elicited by the conventional reversible binding of the hormone with its receptor (Swaneck and Fishman, 1988). By this criterion, one would predict that the suppression of endogenous estradiol secretion and its replacement by ethinyl estrogens, which are principally 2-hydroxylated, would have a beneficial effect on the risk for breast cancer.

Relationships Among Cell Types

There are four critical questions about the way cell types in the breast interact with each other and the possible modulation by oral contraceptives of this interaction in relation to the development of breast cancer:

• To what extent is steroid hormone function in mammary tissue mediated by synthesis and action of extracellular matrix proteins and growth factors (as opposed to a direct effect on specific cells)?

• Are these putative local regulators responsible for heterogeneity of cell morphology, growth potential, and destiny?

• Can estrogen-dependent local growth factor and ECM protein secretion lead to estrogen-independent secretion that results in local autonomy and overgrowth (a clinical observation often made)?

• How relevant are ECM proteins and growth factors to the etiology of breast cancer?

A major theme of clinical observations of mammary cancer is heterogeneity—of cell types, steroid receptor distribution, oncogene expression, in vitro and in vivo responsiveness of antihormones, and prognosis. Additionally, animal studies indicate that different hormones—growth hormone and prolactin, in addition to estrogens—may be of importance in mammary cancer in different species.

Yet another dimension adding complexity in breast physiology is the time domain: ontogenetic, cyclic, pregnancy, lactation, and aging. For example, the nature of stem cells at all of these stages of breast development should be explored. This type of research may provide some clues about the nature of stem cells that give rise to breast cancer in humans, and may be important in the use of experimental models for human breast cancer. These long time periods clearly are characterized by changing serum hormone levels and changing differentiation and growth of mammary tissue per se. The local interactions outlined above may be different in different time domains, thus further increasing complexity.

Receptors

The current concept of the action of any substance that serves as a "signal" to a cell, rather than as a substrate or precursor, is that it must be bound to a specific receptor in the cell membrane, cytoplasm, or nucleus. Three kinds of signals mediated by receptors are relevant to breast physiology: endocrine (hormonal), paracrine (local substance released by neighboring cells), and autocrine (substances secreted by the same cell on which they act).

Breast cells have receptors for estradiol, progesterone, prolactin, cortisol, oxytocin, transforming growth factor β, aldosterone, insulin, epidermal growth factor, placental lactogen, thyroxine, relaxin, growth hormone, calcitonin, insulin-like growth factors I and II, and fibroblast growth factor. This extraordinary diversity of cell receptors for circulating hormones, as well as a large variety of growth factors that may be produced locally, means that investigation of the etiology of transformation in these cells is not a simple matter. In turn, ascribing a possible role of oral contraceptives in such transformation will not be readily proven.

Timing

During the process of development, there are critical periods when a given target tissue can be altered irreversibly by a signal—for example, by a hormone. Once the critical time period has passed the target tissue can no longer be affected. An example of such a critical period is the three- to seven-day period during development of the rodent brain when masculinizing hormones can permanently alter neuronal numbers in the brain. If such masculinization fails to occur during this time, it cannot ever take place. A similar critical period occurs in the human: during myelinization of the brain postnatally, thyroid hormones are critical. If they are not present before about four to six months, the brain is irreversibly stunted and mental retardation results, which cannot be reversed by thyroid hormones. Evidence also indicates that female fetuses of mothers treated with diethylstilbestrol during pregnancy have a higher incidence of vaginal cancer many years later.

Are there any similar critical time periods (e.g., peripubertal or postpubertal) in mammary tissue development when gonadal or pituitary hormones can set some process into motion that leads inexorably to altered development and irreversible differentiation along a given path? In the human breast, certain aspects of development are not initiated until puberty. Could exogenous gonadal steroids administered during the peripubertal period set some event in train that may not be manifested for a number of years, and that would not be initiated by the same steroids administered at less sensitive times to older women?

Effects of Pregnancy and Lactation

The putative protective effects of pregnancy and lactation on breast cancer add several important questions to the research agenda: What is there about pregnancy and lactation that confers protection? Can this be seen in an animal model? Do placental hormones contribute to protection? Beyond these general questions, it has been observed that there is a cyclic difference in both mitogenesis and steroid receptors in the breast when examined using thymidine incorporation and estrogen or progesterone receptor-binding assays, respectively (Anderson et al., 1990). These data suggest additional research questions: What causes increased mitogenesis during the luteal phase? If it is progesterone, what is the mechanism? Is progesterone responsiveness permanently altered by pregnancy and lactation?

Pathological Breast Tissue

Information continues to be needed on both normal and neoplastic tissue. Although the physiology of the breast is relatively well understood, there is still no useful understanding of the transformation from benign to malignant breast epithelium. Pathologists have used biopsy material to identify a small subgroup of women at increased risk, but there is no reason to think that the majority of breast cancers arise from this type of background.

Efforts to determine the effect of oral contraceptives on the risk of developing breast cancer should probably focus on the effect of these agents on normal breast tissue. Cystic conditions—in some instances, gross cystic disease—are common during the reproductive years, and although such tissue might be considered abnormal, recent studies do not reveal an increase in breast cancer in such patients. Further studies of cyst fluid should be conducted because cyst fluid constitutes the best available reflection of breast epithelium. A number of mutagens as well as specific growth factors have been described in cyst fluid. Much of this work focuses on early detection, but it can also be used to investigate hormones that are thought to cause epithelial proliferation in the breast. Both the administration and withdrawal of hormones could be investigated because most women with gross cystic disease form additional cysts. More detailed characterization of breast cyst fluid would be beneficial; once this has been done, the effect of oral contraceptives on a wide variety of biological markers (e.g., gross cystic disease fluid protein) could be determined.

Cysts generally appear during the 30s and 40s; thus, there is also a need for tissue that will provide epithelium from younger women. The best source of such tissue would be fibroadenomas, which are most common between the ages of 15 and 25. These tumors are commonplace but have received little study because they are not associated with cancer. Despite the lack of association, however, efforts should be initiated to identify biological markers that might be affected by hormone administration. Because each patient would only be studied once—second fibroadenomas are far less common than second cysts—methods must be developed for repeated epithelial sampling. Induced nipple secretions have been used for such sampling, but the cytology is extremely variable and may reflect shed rather than viable cells. A better method might be fine-needle aspiration, which can be performed repeatedly with minimal discomfort. Currently, it is used routinely in the diagnosis of neoplasms; however, it can also be used to aspirate normal breast epithelial cells. Epithelium sampled by this method has been examined histologically, but biological studies (with and without cultures) are also possible, provided the appropriate markers (either functional or cytological) can be developed, and would cast additional light on the effect of hormones on normal breast epithelium.

The important question concerning oral contraceptives is their effect on normal breast epithelium, as breast cancer has already been studied intensively. Consequently, the committee emphasizes this necessary concentration on the largest gap in our present knowledge: the transformation of benign to malignant epithelium.

Another area that requires new information relates to family history and efforts to identify oral contraceptive users who might be at increased risk. The study of breast cancer should consider tissue-typing techniques that have made it possible, for example, to identify children who will be affected in families with juvenile diabetes. The search for linkage in breast cancer families is an active field, and improved techniques (i.e., analysis of linkage using polymorphic DNA probes) are now available. These methods should make it possible to better define the genetic makeup of the small group of women with a relatively high risk of breast cancer as a result of specific family history of the disease.

Carcinoma of the breast presents a variable histological appearance, but current classification systems place almost 90 percent of all breast cancers in the invasive (or infiltrating) ductal category. Foote and Stewart described invasive lobular carcinoma—the last new histological subgroup—in 1941; a miscellaneous collection of unusual breast cancers has been recognized for at least 50 years. The largest group would be medullary cancers, but colloid (or mucinous), adenoid cystic, papillary, tubular, and even cancers with carcinoid features or squamous and osseous metaplasia have also been noted. Lobular carcinoma in situ and hyperplasia with atypia also fall into this category. Unlike other cancers induced by carcinogens, no new histological type of breast cancer can be tied to the introduction of oral contraceptives. However, there has been no systematic examination of the rare cancers and use of the pill, and even more important, no study of certain benign lesions associated with increased risk.

A final point relates to the deposition of calcium in the breast. The presence of calcification signals in situ breast cancer on screening mammograms, but only 20 to 30 percent of all breast cancers show microcalcifications. There is no information on the possible role of oral contraceptives in the development of these calcifications.

Oncogenes

Recent studies of the molecular biology of oncogenic transformation (i.e., the process by which a normal cell becomes malignant) have identified various mechanisms. Using animal cell model systems, these studies define various genes, or oncogenes, whose dysregulated expression results in transformation. In some cases, abnormally high levels of specific oncogene products cause transformation. These levels can be achieved in the laboratory for study by amplifying the number of gene copies, by mutating the gene so that it does not respond properly to regulatory elements, or by genetically altering the regulatory elements themselves. This third type of oncogene is dominant because only one allele need be affected to produce abnormally high levels of gene product. In other cases, transformation results when a gene product necessary for normal cellular behavior is missing. Generally, both alleles of the gene must be affected (either deleted or mutated) for the functional gene product to be absent; hence, such genes are often termed recessive oncogenes.

If the effects of estrogens and antiestrogens on mitogenesis and various aspects of breast cell intracellular metabolic pathways are mediated by secondary factors like locally secreted growth factors and extracellular matrix protein production, then any autonomous constitutive secretion of these factors could mediate transformation of an initially estrogen-dependent tumor into an estrogen-independent tumor. This conversion might result from the action of an oncogene.

Because different genes can induce oncogene transformation of animal cells, however, there must be more than one mechanism by which a cell can become malignant. Therefore, it is important to determine which, if any, of the known dominant or recessive oncogenes are actually involved in particular human cancers. To answer this question, human tumor biopsies have been characterized for various genetic aberrations.

Because most biopsies are quite small, technological breakthroughs allowing evaluation of small amounts of nucleic acid have only recently made it possible to study human tumors. Two techniques that have been particularly important are the polymerase chain reaction (PCR) and analysis of restriction fragment length polymorphisms (RFLPs). PCR is a method by which any known gene sequence can be specifically amplified so that as few as 10 to 100 copies of a specific sequence can be detected. RFLP analysis allows researchers to distinguish between two alleles of a given gene because of small variations in DNA fragment size that are detected as differences in migration through acrylamide gels after cleavage with site-specific DNAases. One can deduce that a given allele is missing when one fragment is absent from the gel.

Two generalizations are emerging from these molecular characterizations of cancer biopsies that may be relevant to the problem of identifying a possible role for oral contraceptives in the etiology of breast cancer. First, it is clear that the molecular lesions associated with cancers differ depending on the organ of origin. For example, some of the molecular lesions found in colon cancers and certain lung cancers are not detected in breast cancers. This observation provides evidence at the molecular level for the conclusion that different etiologic factors may be responsible for these three common human cancers. Second, among breast cancers there is a great deal of heterogeneity in the types of genetic lesions detected, which suggests that breast cancer may be more than one disease.

Molecular Changes Associated with Human Breast Cancer

Activated ras Mutations

The products of *ras* oncogenes are functionally and structurally similar to the G-proteins. G-proteins normally act by transmitting proliferative signals initiated by extracellular hormones and growth factors. They bind guanine nucleotides and mediate signal transduction through effectors such as adenylate cyclase. Certain mutations in G-proteins induce autonomous activity by inactivating control regions of the protein; these mutations cause loss of cellular growth capability. *ras* is the only one of the G-protein family that has been extensively studied in human cancers. There are three *ras* genes, Kl-*ras*, Ha-*ras* and N-*ras*. Mutations at codons 12, 13, or 61 are known to activate each of these *ras* genes, resulting in transformation of various cell types (for reviews, see Milburn et al., 1990; Bos, 1989).

The overall incidence of *ras* activation in human cancer has been estimated at 10 to 15 percent. This figure is much higher, however, for specific solid tumors such as adenocarcinomas of the lung (50 percent) and gastrointestinal tract (40 percent), or acute myeloid leukemias. In contrast, *ras* activation is rarely seen in either primary or metastatic breast cancer. Thus, it is unlikely that *ras* activation by gene mutation has any significant role in the initiation of metastatic progression of human breast cancer in vivo. These negative findings are significant in at least two regards. First, they provide evidence of etiologic differences between spontaneous human breast tumors and carcinogen-induced rat models of breast cancer, which have a high incidence of *ras* mutations. Second, they illustrate the molecular biological differences between breast adenocarcinomas and morphologically similar adenocarcinomas of the lung and gastrointestinal tract, which have a high incidence of *ras* mutations.

Overexpression of Tyrosine Kinases

The G-proteins are one example of signal transducers; another common mechanism of signal transduction involves kinases and phosphatases. Protein kinases and phosphatases add or remove phosphate either from serine and threonine residues or from tyrosine residues. Phosphorylation affects the enzymatic activity of a variety of proteins. Many growth factor receptors function as tyrosine kinases. They normally become transiently activated by binding a growth factor; mutations in their transmembrane domains, however, can result in constitutive activity.

In breast cancer, there has been no evidence to date of activating mutations in the transmembrane domains of tyrosine kinase growth factor receptors. Yet abnormal cell growth may also result from overexpression of normal growth factor receptors. Three related tyrosine kinase transmembrane proteins are expressed at increased levels in breast cancer: the epidermal growth factor, or EGF, receptor, the receptor-like product of the *erb*B-2 oncogene, and the product of a recently described gene, *erb*B-3.

The EGF receptor is a 170-kilodalton (kD) transmembrane glycoprotein, which is found on many epithelial cell types. It also binds transforming growth factor alpha (TGF-α), which results in a growth stimulatory effect similar to that observed with EGF. In patients whose breast cancers are negative for estrogen receptor, a high level of EGF receptors is associated with poor prognosis (Huebner et al., 1988), but this issue is still controversial (Foekens et al., 1989). In breast cancers, the cause of EGF receptor overexpression is unknown; only rarely is overexpression caused by EGF receptor gene amplification.

The *erb*B-2 gene (also known as *neu* or *her*-2) is amplified in approximately 10 to 30 percent of breast carcinomas and also in adenocarcinomas of salivary gland, stomach, and ovary. *erb*B-2 is structurally related to the EGF receptor; hence, its gene product is thought to be a growth factor, but its ligand is unknown. Some investigators have shown that *erb*B-2 amplification and protein overexpression correlate with poor prognosis; others have found no such correlation. The evidence for association of *erb*B overexpression with poor prognosis is stronger in patients with lymph node metastases than in node-negative patients.

Much less is known about the role in breast cancers of *erb*B-3, a third member of the *erb* family. It was identified because it is homologous to the EGF receptor gene and to *erb*B-2. Sequence analysis of the cDNA predicts that it encodes a 148-kD transmembrane polypeptide. Like the other members of this family, overexpression of *erb*B-3 occurs in a percentage of breast cancers.

Amplification of int-2 and myc

There are four known *int* genes, which are defined as the sites of common integration of the mouse mammary tumor virus genome. Their sequences fall into two groups: *int*-1 and *int*-2. Although the two groups have no sequence similarity, both are implicated in mouse mammary tumorigenesis and are essential in early embryogenesis.

int-1 related genes are not amplified, translocated, or even expressed in human breast cancer. In contrast, the *int*-2 gene is amplified in 15 percent of breast cancers. It is unlikely, however, that the *int*-2 gene itself is important in breast cancer. Whenever gene amplification occurs, the gene that confers a selective advantage is coamplified, together with 100 to 1,000 kilobases of surrounding DNA. The *int*-2 gene is usually coamplified with certain other genes that have been implicated in human cancer, including *hst*, *bcl*-1, and *sea*. In a minority of breast cancers, *bcl*-1 is the only gene of the cluster that is amplified; in some cases, none of the three genes is expressed. There is hence some question of which gene is the driving force in the amplicon, and it has been hypothesized that an as yet unknown gene in the region, when amplified, confers a selective growth advantage on breast cancers.

Much less work has been done on the role of c-*myc* in breast cancer. C-*myc* is a nuclear protein that may be involved in transcriptional regulation of other genes important for cellular growth control. Amplification of the c-*myc* gene has been observed in approximately 5 to 30 percent of breast cancers.

Deletions of Genes

Researchers are increasingly aware that mutations resulting in loss of function play an important role in the pathogenesis of human malignancies. Deletion of one allele, measured by loss of heterozygosity for restriction fragment length polymorphism, is thought to unmask mutations in the corresponding normal allele. Thus, it is thought that recessive oncogenes are located in chromosomal regions showing a high incidence of allele loss.

In breast cancer, investigators report nonrandom loss of heterozygosity for a number of chromosomal loci. The frequency of loss of heterozygosity ranged from approximately 50 percent for chromosome 17p, to 20 to 30 percent for regions on chromosomes 1q, 3p, 11p, 13q, 17q, and 18q. Moreover, it has been suggested that deletions at several loci tend to occur within the same tumors.

At some of the deleted chromosomal loci, researchers have tentatively identified the recessive oncogene involved. The target for loss on chromosome 13q is thought to be the *Rb* gene, which was originally isolated as the recessive oncogene that causes retinoblastoma. The *Rb* gene encodes a protein that is thought to be involved in cell cycle regulation. The region deleted on chromosome 17p includes the p53 gene, which encodes a protein that binds to DNA as a homodimer. In vivo, it may function by binding to and thereby inactivating the suppressor gene products.

RESEARCH MODELS

To address the basic biological questions in the relationship of breast cancer and oral contraceptives, appropriate model systems need to be developed. A recurrent issue in biological research is whether findings in studies of subprimates are predictive of similar findings in humans. Animal models (see Appendix D) have been valuable in studies of breast cancer; in both rodents and dogs, investigators have shown that estrogens can increase the rate of mammary cancer. However, there may be fundamental differences in overall endocrine physiology among various species that preclude direct extrapolation of data from animal models to humans. For example, one pituitary factor, prolactin, is necessary for production of estrogen-induced tumors in mice, whereas a related but different pituitary factor, growth hormone, serves the same function in beagle dogs (see Appendix D). Thus, it is possible that species-specific effects of exogenous steroids such as oral contraceptives will be of primary importance with regard to induction of mammary cancers.

Because many types of physiological studies are impossible in humans, there is a continuing need for animal studies. The conclusions from these studies, however, must be reinforced using human tissue and cells. Consequently, relevant in vitro human systems are essential. There are four types of in vitro human systems currently being used: (1) established tumor cell lines, (2) short-term mammary epithelial cell cultures, (3) organ cultures, and (4) athymic mice. Although tremendous progress has been made using these systems, they are still far from adequate for detecting slight increases in transformation or subtle effects on differentiation. Because it is likely that the effects of many exogenous agents such as oral contraceptives will be small and subtle with respect to cancer induction, further development and refinement of appropriate culture systems are essential. Therefore, the committee recommends that a sustained, long-term basic research effort to develop and refine appropriate culture systems is warranted. Furthermore, the specific steroids contained in oral contraceptives should be studied using these systems. Finally, it is crucially important to refer to whole-animal in vivo studies to verify that in vitro findings have relevance to the whole animal.

Breast Cancer Cell Lines

Breast cancer established cell lines are valuable because they provide a readily available source of proliferating cells with infinite growth potential. In many cases, these lines retain in vivo properties, thereby providing useful substrates for many important physiological studies. For example, much information on the cellular biology of estrogen receptors has been gathered because some breast cancer cell lines retain estrogen receptors in culture. This readily available source of estrogen receptor-positive cells permitted extensive characterization of the mechanisms by which estrogen receptors control gene expression (for a review, see Dickson and Lippman, 1987). Studies using these cell lines have also been directly useful in the clinic because the cell lines support more rapid, detailed characterization of potential estrogen receptor inhibitors, such as tamoxifen.

Although established cell lines derived from breast carcinomas have provided tools for many informative and important studies, the interpretation of this information must take into account the limitations of such cell lines. Normal human mammary cells do not develop into established cell lines. Furthermore, the existing breast cancer cell lines represent only a small subset of breast cancer cells because (1) only occasional cells within a given tumor survive as the cell line, and (2) only rare breast cancer specimens develop into cell lines.

To develop a cell line, the tumor cells are usually held in a maintenance state for prolonged periods, sometimes months, before a cell population emerges that can grow continuously in culture. During the initial period, most of the carcinoma cells obtained from the malignant tissue proliferate a few times and then undergo a phenomenon, or "crisis," in which most of them stop proliferating, deteriorate, and disappear from the culture vessel. The cell line subsequently emerges from a subpopulation of the remaining cells.

Furthermore, only a small number of breast cancer specimens, most of which are derived from metastatic lesions, contain a cell subpopulation capable of proliferating subsequent to crisis. Even among effusion metastases, the most widely studied type of metastatic lesion, less than 10 percent actually develop cell lines. Among primary breast cancers, the frequency of cell line development is much lower, reaching incidences of approximately 1 in 200 cases.

The ability to survive crisis and become an immortalized cell line is not random, either in relation to culture technique or to tumor progression. In one study (Smith et al., 1987), the properties in culture of breast cancer effusion metastases, obtained over approximately two years from the same patient, were examined. Despite repeated attempts with cryopreserved cells, only the last specimen reproducibly exhibited immortality in culture; the first two specimens grew initially but failed to survive crisis. Each specimen was unique in morphology, growth properties, and oncogene aberrations, although karyotypic markers indicated a common origin. The observation that the last effusion metastasis could develop reproducibly into a cell line when prior malignant effusions from the same patient could not suggests that the capacity for infinite life in culture depends on inherent changes in the biological phenotype of the tumor rather than on irreproducible vagaries of cell culture. This study, together with numerous observations that metastatic specimens develop into cell lines much more commonly than primary breast cancers, indicates that the capacity for infinite life in vitro results from a phenotype that is usually acquired by breast cancer cells at a late stage of malignant progression.

Short-term Culture of Normal Mammary Epithelium

Studies on breast cancer cell lines cannot address many of the relevant questions related to the potential link of oral contraceptives and breast cancer. Therefore, it will be critical to develop in vitro model systems that use normal human mammary epithelium.

There are two main sources for culturing normal mammary epithelial cells: breast milk and reduction mammoplasties. Large numbers of epithelial cells can be obtained from milk, particularly during early stages of weaning, when the mammary ducts and alveoli are involuting and being sloughed into the luminal contents (Russo et al., 1975; Kirkland et al., 1979). The epithelial cells derived from milk have the advantage of being free of fibroblast contamination, although they generally grow less well than those isolated from reduction mammoplasties.

To isolate cells from reduction mammoplasties, researchers must separate the cells from massive amounts of connective tissue and fat by enzymatic digestion. The epithelial cells, which are connected by junctional complexes that are insensitive to these enzymes, remain as clumps; the stromal fibroblasts and connective tissues are dissociated to single cells. The epithelial cells can then easily be isolated free of fibroblasts by sedimentation at unit gravity or by filtration through nylon mesh filters. This technique also isolates capillary endothelium, but the endothelial cells do not grow in the media formulations developed for the epithelium.

Mammary epithelial cells proliferate in a variety of culture conditions, including collagen coating of the culture surface, the presence of various growth factors such as epidermal growth factor and cholera toxin, reduced calcium concentrations, or conditioned media from specific cell lines. The cells also grow to some extent in a variety of completely defined media containing high-density lipoproteins, extracellular matrix, various hormones, and growth factors.

A number of criteria have been used to verify the epithelial origin of the cultured cells. Cultured breast cells have a typical cuboidal morphology and form secretory domes and ductlike, three-dimensional ridges at confluence. Ultrastructurally, the cells show junctional complexes and evidence of secretory activity. They also have a distinctive punctate pattern of cell-associated fibronectin and express epithelial membrane antigens as defined by antibodies raised to milk-fat globules. The epithelial origin of the mammary epithelial cells has been further verified using antibodies to cytokeratins, the intermediate filament proteins, characteristic of epithelial cells (for reviews, see Osborn and Weber, 1983; Taylor-Papadimitriou and Lane, 1987).

Although the epithelial nature of cultured mammary cells has been clearly established, the type of mammary epithelium being cultured is controversial. In vivo, normal mammary epithelium is organized into ducts and alveoli, and within the ducts, there are both basal (sometimes referred to as myoepithelial) and luminal epithelial cells. The different types of epithelium have not been successfully separated prior to culture. After culture, it has been difficult to identify which cells were derived from the different epithelial components. In vivo, basal cells of the mammary ducts are positive for the cell surface marker CALLA (Gusterson et al., 1986), and for cytokeratin 14 (Dairkee et al., 1985), a member of the cytokeratin family. Luminal cells express epithelial antigens derived from milk fat, and other cytokeratin markers (for a review, see Taylor-Papadimitriou et al., 1977). When reduction mammoplasty cells are cultured, all of the cells are positive for cytokeratin 14 and CALLA, suggesting that basal epithelial cells are preferentially grown in culture. Many of the same cells, however, are also positive for a luminal antigen (Dairkee et al., 1986). Therefore, one cannot rule out the possibility that luminal dedifferentiation occurs after culture. An excellent analysis of numerous markers of mammary epithelial differentiation in culture (Petersen and van Deurs, 1988) concluded that the mammary differentiation phenotype is plastic and can be modulated by growth factors and other media components.

Because steroid hormones are intimately involved in mammary gland differentiation, it is critical that future studies concentrate on developing better culture systems for maintaining the differentiated state to allow distinguishing among ductal, alveolar, basal, and luminal epithelium. Only then will it be possible to explore in vitro the critical research questions that relate to the actions of oral contraceptives on normal breast tissue function.

Organ Culture

In vitro cell culture has been invaluable for studying the effects of various stimuli directly on synthesis and secretion of many cell products. Usually such cultures contain predominantly one cell type, which enhances their usefulness for examining specificity of stimulus and response. But this simple system has been proved inadequate to examine regulation when two or more cell types communicate with each other and act as a coordinated system. For example, research has shown that, in developing gonadal steroid target tissues, the steroid receptor develops first in the stromal tissue and the steroid acts on the epithelial cell by means of a local signal generated by the stroma. Such cell-cell interactions occur in all organs. Increasingly, in vitro systems using pieces of organs that contain several cell types are being used as more "normal" models to examine putative regulators of synthesis, secretion, and morphology. These breast-tissue organ-culture systems must be explored more fully than in the past, however, particularly in light of increased evidence of the importance of locally secreted growth factors and extracellular matrix proteins in determining epithelial cell function. It is possible that local misregulation is actually the mechanism by which transformation of specific cells takes place. One negative aspect of organ culture is that the heterogeneity of cells means that certain effects need to be measured in situ on the cells, in addition to measuring factors released into the medium.

Nude Mouse Model

The athymic nude mouse model system is an immunologically incompetent mouse that does not reject tissue from other species. Normal mammary epithelium can grow in cleared fat pads of nude mice and forms normal ductal structures. Some breast cancer cell lines form tumors readily in these animals. Hence, the nude mouse provides a useful "in vivo/in vitro" system to study factors that contribute to tumor growth. Athymic mice do not secrete much estrogen because their ovaries undergo premature failure and thus exogenous estrogen must be given for tumor growth of human breast cell lines. This exogenous estrogen can act locally—that is, directly on the breast tumor cells. The model has also shown that mutagenesis by estrogen of human breast cancer cells can be potentiated by cotransplants of a pituitary cell line, GH3 cells, suggesting that a pituitary factor (not GH or prolactin) may also be necessary for this process (Dembinski et al., 1985).

The usefulness of the nude mouse is that the animal itself provides the "culture milieu" for its transplanted tissue, and this natural medium is renewed appropriately by the circulatory system. These culture conditions may simulate the intact mammary tissue better than in vitro conditions. Furthermore, given the mouse's low endogenous estrogen levels, this model may be valuable for studying the effects of cyclic administration of various oral contraceptives on normal mammary epithelium.

SUMMARY AND CONCLUSIONS

Although recent studies of mammary gland development, physiology, cell biology, and molecular biology have increased our knowledge considerably, there are no definitive answers as yet that enable us to understand, in all of its aspects, the biological etiology of breast cancer. A number of leads should be followed. Does the 16α-hydroxysteroid metabolic pathway lead to production of a hormone metabolite that binds the estrogen receptor more tightly than normal, leading to abnormal or enhanced gene products? Do exogenous estrogens regulate this pathway or act differently than endogenous estrogens? Are local growth factors and the newly detected extracellular matrix proteins, such as tenascin, important in the etiology of breast cancer? If not, can they serve at least as markers of the stage or etiology of the disease? Are oncogenes always involved ultimately in breast cancer (regardless of the initial insult)? Will the different oncogenes that are possibly involved act through the same final common pathway to cause transformation? Questions such as these, and many others, need to be vigorously pursued in a multidisciplinary setting to expand our understanding of breast biology in a way that will be relevant to the etiology of breast cancer.

A number of different genetic aberrations have been seen in breast cancers, but in each instance, the lesions are found only in a proportion of all such cancers. Preliminary observations suggest that some lesions may be coordinately expressed; thus, it may be possible to define subsets of breast cancer by their constellations of molecular aberrations. Breast cancers are unusual in that tumors of similar histology and staging may have widely varying clinical courses. This variability and the existence of molecular subsets suggest that breast cancer may be more than one disease, each with differing etiologies. If so, insights into putative etiologic agents—for example, oral contraceptives—may be acquired by determining whether their use is correlated with specific molecular breast cancer subsets.

With respect to oral contraceptive formulations (see Appendix C), four questions emerge as immediate research priorities: Do individual variations in blood levels in ethinyl estradiol and the progestin component of oral contraceptives affect the risk of breast cancer? What are the effects of the progestin component of oral contraceptives in modulating estrogen action? Do the inherent androgenic or antiestrogenic properties of different oral contraceptive formulations affect normal breast tissue response? How will the overall estrogen dominance of the new oral contraceptives affect breast tissue response?

Cancerous breast tissue has been well studied. For the 1990s, intense focus on normal rather than neoplastic epithelium is warranted. Because the significant issue concerning oral contraceptives is their effect on normal breast epithelium, the committee emphasizes the importance of concentrating on the largest gap in present knowledge: the transformation of benign to malignant epithelium.

4

Information for Users of the Pill
and Health Care Providers

Oral contraceptives are widely used and have been the object of more studies and data gathering than any other pharmaceutical preparation. Nonetheless, widespread consumer confusion prevails. A 1985 poll on consumer perception conducted for the American College of Obstetricians and Gynecologists revealed that (1) 75 percent of women believed that the pill carried substantial health risks, (2) 33 percent believed that the pill caused cancer, and (3) 66 percent believed that taking the pill was more dangerous than bearing a child. In light of these findings, the public must be kept better informed, and health care providers must keep themselves informed of the current status of the health benefit/risk ratio relative to the use of oral contraceptives.

BENEFITS AND RISKS OF ORAL CONTRACEPTIVES

Benefits

The pill is the most effective, reversible contraceptive in widespread use today. In the United States, it is a major factor in preventing unintended pregnancy and induced abortion.

Aside from their extraordinary effectiveness as contraceptives, oral contraceptives have been shown to have numerous noncontraceptive benefits (Table 4-1). The pill usually regulates menstrual cycles and reduces menstrual flow, thus preventing iron-deficiency anemia and

TABLE 4-1 Well-established Major Protective Effects of Oral Contraceptives (OC) by Problem or Condition, United Kingdom or United States

Problem or Condition Protected Against	Relative Risk Current Use	Past Use	Influenced by Duration of Use	Influenced by OC Formulation
Menstrual problems[a]	0.75	1.0	No	Yes—protection decreases with "low-dose" pills
Iron-deficiency anemia[a]	0.75	1.0	No	Unknown
Benign breast cysts[a]	0.5	1.0	Yes—protection increases as duration increases	Yes—protection increases as progestin increases
Pelvic inflammatory disease[a]	0.5	1.0	Unknown	Unknown
Functional ovarian cysts[a]	0.25	1.0	No	Probably not
Epithelial ovarian cancer[b]	0.5	0.5	Yes—protection increases as duration increases	Probably not
Endometrial cancer[b]	0.5	0.5	Yes—protection increases as duration increases	Probably not

[a]Based on hospital admissions data.
[b]Based on incidence data.

SOURCE: Adapted from M. P. Vessey, "The Jephcott Lecture, 1989: An Overview of the Benefits and Risks of Combined Oral Contraceptives," in *Oral Contraceptives and Breast Cancer*, R. D. Mann, ed. (Park Ridge, N.J.: The Parthenon Publishing Group, 1990).

reducing hospital admissions for problems related to menorrhagia. Evidence also indicates that the risk of pelvic inflammation decreases in women taking the pill. (Some recent work suggests, however, that the pill is associated with an increased risk of chlamydial infection, although a clear association has not been established in a prospective study.) Use of the pill is associated with decreased risk of ovarian tumors, both benign and malignant; in addition, the risk of endometrial carcinoma begins to decline after one year of oral contraceptive use. Protection against ovarian and endometrial malignancy is greatest in nulliparous women. The risk of ectopic pregnancy and its adverse effects on reproductive health are also decreased in pill users (because most oral contraceptives prevent ovulation, which, of course, precludes pregnancy, ectopic or otherwise).

Risks

In the history of unraveling the side effects of the pill, the first described complication of oral contraceptives was related to cardiovascular problems (Table 4-2). The relative risk of venous thrombosis for current users is an estimated 5 times that for nonusers, with a low absolute risk. It seems that venous thrombosis and pulmonary embolism are related mostly to the pill's estrogenic component, whereas other cardiovascular complications relate primarily to the progestin component.

Myocardial infarction is rare in young women, and no deaths have been reported in users of the pill who are under 25 years of age, even among smokers. Episodes of acute hypertension are almost nonexistent in users of pill formulations that contain less than 50 μg of estrogen.

Both thrombotic and hemorrhagic stroke have been described and can be identified in 5 to 10 percent of all deaths in women who were using oral contraceptives at the time of their death. Recent studies have shown that, with the exception of subarachnoid hemorrhage, there is no increase in risk of stroke among nonsmokers who use oral contraceptives. Careful patient screening and physician sensitivity to premonitory symptoms, especially headaches, should decrease the risk. There is no substantially increased risk of stroke among former users of steroid contraception.

An association has been observed between oral contraceptives and the occurrence of rare hepatocellular adenomas. These tumors are benign but can be associated with pill use (Table 4-2). For hepatocellular carcinoma, which is also rare (i.e., approximately 1 case per 100,000 women in the United States), pill users face a risk three times that of nonusers.

CURRENT CONTROVERSY

It is estimated that one American woman in nine develops breast cancer sometime in her life, thus reducing by 25 percent her chances of surviving the next five years. The major correlate of risk is a woman's age. Breast cancer is rarely evident in the mid-teens. By age 30-34, the annual occurrence is 30 cases per 100,000 women; by age 70-74, the rate has increased to 424 cases per 100,000 women (1986 data; see

TABLE 4-2 Well-established Major Adverse Effects of Oral
Contraceptives (OC), United Kingdom or United States

Adverse Effect[a]	Relative Risk		Influenced by Duration of Use	Influenced by OC Formulation
	Current Use	Past Use		
Acute myocardial infarction[b]	2	1	Probably not	Probably yes— risk increases as estrogen and progestin increase
Thrombotic stroke[b]	5	1	Probably not	Unknown
Hemorrhagic stroke[b]	1.5	1.5	Probably not	Unknown
Venous thromboembolism[b]	5	1	No	Probably yes— risk increases as estrogen increases
Hepatocellular adenoma[c]	50		Yes—risk increases as duration increases	Yes—risk increases, with "high-dose" pills
Hepatocellular carcinoma[d]	3		Yes—risk increases as duration increases	Unknown

[a]Data are not included on hypertension because the adverse consequences of this condition are expressed in terms of myocardial infarction or stroke.
[b]Based on data for hospital admissions or deaths.
[c]Based on incidence data.
[d]Based on incidence and mortality data.

SOURCE: Adapted from M. P. Vessey, "The Jephcott Lecture, 1989: An Overview of the Benefits and Risks of Combined Oral Contraceptives," in *Oral Contraceptives and Breast Cancer*, R. D. Mann, ed. (Park Ridge, N.J.: The Parthenon Publishing Group, 1990).

Table 1-7). After age and nationality, the major risk factors for breast cancer are (1) early age at menarche, (2) late age at menopause, (3) nulliparity, (4) late age at first full-term pregnancy, (5) breast cancer in first-degree relatives, and (6) elevated postmenopausal weight.

Despite the effectiveness of the pill as a contraceptive agent, its numerous noncontraceptive benefits, and evidence that the cumulative risk of breast cancer through at least age 45 appears to have no relationship to pill use, significant uncertainty and concern remain. Several recent epidemiological studies restricted to women under the age of 45 have raised the possibility of an adverse effect from long-term oral contraceptive use before a first full-term pregnancy. Given the fact that the majority of pill users in this country are now younger women who have not yet had such a pregnancy and who take the pill for extended periods, this concern and the recognition that further studies are needed seem most appropriate.

At present, it is unknown if, in fact, risk of breast cancer increases in younger pill users who have used the pill for a long time—whether or not they have had their first full-term pregnancy. Epidemiological research studies must be structured to answer this question. If such studies do show increased risk, several questions must be answered: (1) What is the magnitude of the risk? (2) How long does it persist? ·and (3) Given the overall benefit/risk ratio of the pill, is its continued use warranted?

PRESCRIBING PROBLEMS

Health professionals must provide concise, accurate counsel to their patients based on a clear, current understanding of the balance of benefits and risks of pill use and the user's health and sociocultural status. The absolute contraindications to pill use, as they appear in the patient package insert, are: undiagnosed abnormal genital bleeding; presence or history of breast or liver malignancy; thromboembolic disorders; cerebrovascular disease; myocardial infarction; known or suspected estrogen-dependent neoplasia; and known or suspected pregnancy.

Additionally, a number of factors place a patient at a potentially higher risk for complications with the use of oral contraceptives. A list of these factors appears in the package insert, as follows: age over 40; heavy smoking over age 35; family history of premature death from cardiovascular disease; hypertension; abnormal metabolic conditions; gestational diabetes; hyperlipidemia; severe migraine; and chronic liver disease. In 1989, an advisory committee of the Food and Drug Administration recommended removal of any upper age limit.

It is important to note that practitioners are obliged to provide women with information about the current state of ambiguity regarding the relationship between oral contraceptives and breast cancer. Some women will be distressed by this lack of a clear picture and will find it difficult to incorporate this uncertainty into their decision-making process. They should be encouraged, however, to look at the total picture—especially the known benefits and risks of oral contraceptives, as well as the known benefits and risks of other birth control methods, and the risks of unintended pregnancy—in making their choices about contraception. For many women, the convenience and dependability of the pill will continue to outweigh worries about a possible link to breast cancer. For others, this possible link will provide motivation to use another method. Adequate information and supportive counseling will help each woman sort through her own, unique situation.

Although the possibility exists that younger pill users may have increased risk of breast cancer prior to first full-term birth, based on the current state of knowledge as to the benefit/risk ratio of pill use, the committee recommends no fundamental change in prescribing practice for oral contraceptives at this time.

5

Policy Issues and Recommendations

Efforts to untangle the relationship, if any, between current and future oral contraceptives and breast cancer will be long, slow, and relatively expensive. They will also be tightly linked to whatever progress is made in the overall understanding of the pathogenesis of the disease, including markers of susceptibility and response to oral contraceptive exposure. In view of the high costs, in human and financial terms, associated with a continuously rising incidence of breast cancer and the potential importance of any possible relationship with oral contraceptives, the committee offers recommendations that address four policy areas:

- maintaining surveillance;
- developing a broader array of contraceptives;
- assessing knowledge for application in clinical practice; and
- filling gaps in biological and epidemiological knowledge.

Taken together, the committee's recommendations call for a new, more explicit level of planning, investment, and commitment—directed toward the study of breast cancer in general and its relationship to steroid hormones—in particular, oral contraceptives.

MAINTAINING SURVEILLANCE

With oral contraceptives in widespread use, epidemiologists must maintain appropriate surveillance throughout at least the next 20 to 40 years to follow the effects of current formulations of the pill, when used from an early age, on breast cancer risk. As current formulations are likely to be the highest doses used over the period, the assessment of their effects cannot be cut short. To date, the cohort studies performed in the United Kingdom have been among the best and have yielded the most information. European and Scandinavian populations may continue to be important resources for surveillance: some are particularly stable, and several have prescription records of high quality and long duration. Also, some oral contraceptive formulations bound for the United States are already in use in Europe. In the United States, members of large, stable health maintenance organizations may be similarly important resources for surveillance.

Plans are already being formulated to establish sound Medicare data bases and cohorts to permit studies of the effectiveness of medical interventions (Heithoff and Lohr, 1990). Consideration should be given to ways in which linkages with the new Medicare data bases could be used to explore the influence of earlier oral contraceptive use on breast cancer incidence among older, postmenopausal women.

The Surveillance, Epidemiology, and End Results (SEER) Program monitors community-wide cancer incidence among women of all races. These registries are the nation's resource for epidemiological studies. They must maintain and, if necessary, expand their capacity to support the necessary epidemiological studies of the influence of oral contraceptive use on breast cancer incidence among U.S. women of different races and cultures.

The surveillance that needs to continue to cover oral contraceptive use and all reproductive cancers will be particularly demanding. The Cancer and Steroid Hormones (CASH) Study conducted by the Centers for Disease Control cost approximately $13.7 million. Even this sizable study, however, was not large enough to answer questions concerning the risk of breast cancer in subgroups of users. Future studies must (1) involve many thousands of cases and controls to permit statistically valid analyses of subgroups of users (e.g., individuals who used the pill prior to their first pregnancy), and (2) follow sufficient numbers of women for many years to measure how long any possible effect persists after discontinuing oral contraceptive use. These are studies of daunting size that cannot be conducted on an ad hoc basis. Nevertheless, they must be undertaken—and the necessary resources must be set aside to conduct them—to protect the health of American women.

Cooperative Research

European and North American research data on breast cancer and oral contraceptives have been complementary. There is enough variation in both exposure to oral contraceptives and opportunities for surveillance among the countries gathering data that a coordinated future research plan offers worldwide benefits. For example, if the prospective study by the United Kingdom Royal College of General Practitioners were continued, it might throw important light on the duration of any relationship between reproductive cancers and oral contraceptive use, as well as on any possible interaction between use of the pill and breast cancer in women over 50 years of age. If the Royal College researchers and U.S. investigators were to reanalyze their data and pool their results, they could well realize the complementary potential of their studies.

Surveillance Requirements of the Food and Drug Administration

At present, a considerable imbalance exists between the investment required by the Food and Drug Administration (FDA) in premarketing testing of a new drug and the investment made in postmarketing surveillance. Indeed, although FDA regulates premarketing testing in great detail, it has never required specific postmarketing studies by the manufacturers of oral contraceptives. Yet, the information from premarketing testing alone cannot answer questions about rare adverse or beneficial effects, such as those central to any consideration of oral contraceptives and reproductive cancers.

The Phase III clinical trials of new drugs required by FDA for new drug application approval cost between $10 and $30 million per trial and are paid for by the developers, or manufacturers. In the special case of contraceptives, where industry is sometimes reluctant to take a leadership role (National Research Council/Institute of Medicine, 1990), part or all of the cost may be met by the federal government (e.g., the National Institutes of Health [NIH] or the Agency for International Development [AID]). All of the postmarketing surveillance of oral contraceptives that has been conducted thus far has been supported by foundations, by NIH or AID, or by the European medical research councils. Although postmarketing surveillance is funded at a much lower level than premarketing testing, it has produced practically all the key clinical information that has led to safer preparations (e.g., low estrogen dose pills) and greater selectivity in use (e.g., avoiding use of the pill by women who smoke). Therefore, the committee recommends that the FDA consider premarketing and postmarketing requirements as an integrated whole and devise ways of spreading the investment already required by manufacturers, and ultimately paid for by users, in such a way as to maximize the information on safety that will result.

DEVELOPING A BROADER ARRAY OF CONTRACEPTIVES

The success and popularity of oral contraceptives as a means of avoiding conception are both a tribute to their efficacy and a reflection of the paucity of effective alternative means, particularly for young women. The committee underscores the urgent need for research and development of a broader array of contraceptives (see NRC/IOM, 1990), including more effective barrier methods and nonsteroidal methods. It is not feasible to wait for resolution of the uncertainty about oral contraceptives as a potential risk factor for breast cancer before energizing research and development on alternative methods of contraception. In the face of uncertainty, those couples wishing to eschew oral contraceptives in favor of other methods of contraception must be served—and sooner, not later. Unless immediate steps are taken to develop a broader array of safe and effective contraceptives, the choice of contraceptives in the United States in the next century will be the same as it is today (NRC/IOM, 1990).

It is worth noting that when new, systemically active methods of contraception are introduced, they will be surrounded by some of the same uncertainty about long-term effects that was first associated with oral contraceptive use. It will take many years of careful study to acquire as much information about a completely new method of contraception as is now available about oral contraceptives.

ASSESSING KNOWLEDGE FOR APPLICATION IN CLINICAL PRACTICE

Health care providers and patients are compelled to make clinical decisions about the use of oral contraceptives based on the best knowledge available to them. The committee finds that, at the outset of the 1990s, the best available knowledge about oral contraceptives and breast cancer does not support any fundamental change in clinical practice with respect to the use of oral contraceptives. This finding is subject to an important caveat: the knowledge base must be reassessed at regular intervals, in light of new research results (e.g., those forthcoming from the World Health Organization and the National

Cancer Institute). The committee recommends that, three years hence, and at regular intervals thereafter, an NIH consensus conference reassess recommendations for oral contraceptive use based on reevaluation of up-to-date information about the relationship between oral contraceptives and breast cancer. Two institutes in particular, the National Institute of Child Health and Human Development and the National Cancer Institute, would be appropriate lead institutes to judge when consensus conferences should be held.

Research results should be periodically assessed for new evidence of short- and long-term safety and carefully analyzed to provide clinicians with current information on the safest oral contraceptive use for younger and older women. There is also a need for continuous improvement of the dissemination of new and existing information about oral contraceptives and breast cancer among health care providers and women who use oral contraceptives. Multiple channels, through which providers and women can receive up-to-date information, must be opened and maintained. These channels include continuing medical education courses, the technical bulletins and other activities of the American College of Obstetricians and Gynecologists and other professional organizations, the activities of state and local health departments, services delivered by the health units of colleges and high schools, and the "one-on-one" contacts so common to the health profession. The committee emphasizes the obligation of health care providers to offer adequate, accurate information to women seeking contraception and to counsel them regarding the current state of ambiguity with respect to the relationship between oral contraceptives and breast cancer. Only then can fully informed choices be made in clinical practice.

FILLING GAPS IN BIOLOGICAL AND EPIDEMIOLOGICAL KNOWLEDGE

The committee believes that a multidisciplinary research approach is necessary to resolve the relationship between oral contraceptives and breast cancer. Research on a broad front could well produce insights that would lead to some reduction in the incidence of breast cancer, in the same way that research throughout the past three decades has led to insights and changes of lifestyle that are today believed to be reducing the incidence of heart disease in America. With no single, "magic bullet" likely to prevent or cure breast cancer, the committee recommends a broad program of expanded studies on breast function and pathophysiology from the perspectives of endocrinology, biochemistry, molecular genetics, nutrition, cytology, and tissue culture.

Basic research in the biology of the breast is identified by the committee as a priority. As one author (McCarty, 1989) notes, "That so much effort has been concentrated on the study of the abnormal with so little knowledge of normal physiology is an aberration. . . . One is struck by the paucity of existing understanding of 'normal' breast development, and the myriad factors influencing the proliferation of normal breast epithelium."

Research is especially needed on the transition from normal to abnormal growth—including, for example, research on the role of local growth factors and newly detected extracellular matrix proteins, estrogen metabolism (e.g., the products of the 16α-hydroxysteroid metabolic pathway), and oncogenes. As basic resources for this research, in vitro model systems that employ normal breast tissue are needed, in which the effects of contraceptive steroids can be directly examined.

Epidemiological research priorities include a large, case-control (retrospective) study with sufficient statistical power to resolve the assessment of small increases in relative risk of breast cancer. One such study is currently being conducted by the National Cancer Institute; it involves primarily women below the age of 45. A study of postmenopausal women—who experience the bulk of breast cancer—is needed to elucidate the effects of both oral contraceptive use alone, and oral contraceptive use followed by hormone replacement therapy. As oral contraceptive formulations and use patterns of the pill change, future case-control studies will be required; the committee has outlined seven strategies that are likely to improve these future studies (see Chapter 2). The launching of appropriate, cost-effective new cohort (prospective) studies is equal in priority to the conduct of case-control studies. There are no substitutes for analytical, observational epidemiological studies in resolving the relationship of oral contraceptives and breast cancer, and great attention should be given to identifying the organizational settings (e.g., health maintenance organizations) in which they can be implemented. Efforts must also be made to establish coordinated international plans (particularly American-British plans) for case-control and cohort studies to monitor the long-term safety of current and widely used new formulations.

Biological markers, as they become more generally available, should be incorporated into epidemiological protocols. Consistent with a multidisciplinary approach to better understanding of the causes of breast cancer, there is a need for research that uses biological markers within the context of epidemiological study designs, using innovative as well as traditional research tactics.

The expensive, complex program of studies necessary to reveal the relationship (if any) between oral contraceptives and breast cancer will inevitably draw on funding from several sources. The cost of such action must be weighed against the sobering costs of inaction: increased suffering and loss of life, the cost of treating breast cancer, and the cost of mammography screening programs, which lead to earlier detection but not to primary prevention. With oral contraceptives now being used by an estimated 10.7 million American women (Mosher and Pratt, 1990), any adverse or beneficial interaction with breast cancer would be highly significant. Furthermore, any proven relationship or, what is equally important, any perceived relationship, would also have a marked effect on contraceptive practice in the United States. This country already has a higher rate of unintended pregnancies than many Western European nations. One in 10 American teenage girls becomes pregnant each year, with abortion a consequence for many. A sudden switch from oral contraceptives to less effective methods—if such a change were based on false interpretation of oral contraceptive risk—would be a public health disaster. Alternatively, if a shift were based on genuine findings, it would require considerable strengthening of family planning services to ensure a smooth transition.

References

Anderson, T. J., S. Battersby, R. J. B. King, and K. Mcpherson. 1990. Breast epithelial responses and steroid receptors during oral contraceptive use. Pp. 363-372 in Oral Contraceptives and Breast Cancer, R. D. Mann, ed. Park Ridge, N.J.: The Parthenon Publishing Group.

Bos, J. L. 1989. ras Oncogenes in human cancer: A review. Cancer Research 49:4682-4689.

Brinton, L. A. 1990. Update of the 1982 study among participants in the Breast Cancer Detection Demonstration Project and plans for a new study. Pp. 207-219 in Oral Contraceptives and Breast Cancer, R. D. Mann, ed. Park Ridge, N.J.: The Parthenon Publishing Group.

The Cancer Letter. 1990. 32% rise in breast cancer diagnosis in 1980s explained by increase in mammography screening. Vol. 16:1-4.

Dairkee, S. H., C. M. Blayney, H. S. Smith, and A. J. Hackett. 1985. Monoclonal antibody that defines human myoepithelium. Proceedings of the National Academy of Sciences USA 82:7409-7413.

Dairkee, S. H., C. M. Blayney, H. S. Smith, and A. J. Hackett. 1986. Concurrent expression of myoepithelial and epithelial markers in cultures of normal human breast analyzed with monoclonal antibodies. Differentiation 32:93-100.

Dawson, D. A. 1990. Trends in oral contraceptive use: Data from the 1987 National Health Interview Survey. Family Planning Perspectives 22:169-172.

Dembinski, T. C., C. K. H. Leung, and R. P. C. Shiu. 1985. Evidence for a novel pituitary factor that potentiates the mitogenic effect of estrogen in human breast cancer cells. Cancer Research 45:3083-3089.

Devesa, S. S., D. T. Silverman, J. L. Young, Jr., E. S. Pollack, C. C. Brown, J. W. Horm, C. L. Percy, M. H. Myers, F. W. McKay, and J. F. Fraumeni, Jr. 1987. Cancer incidence and mortality trends among whites in the United States, 1947-84. Journal of the National Cancer Institute 79:701-770.

Dickson, R. B., and M. E. Lippman. 1987. Estrogenic regulation of growth and polypeptide growth factor secretion in human breast carcinoma. Endocrinology Reviews 8:29-43.

El Shafei, M., S. Varakamin, S. Basnayake, I. L. Diop, E. O. Otolorin, L. Rosero, R. Molina, L. Nunez, O. de la Cueva, F. E. Riphagen, G. S. Grubb, K. S. Hilton, and M. Potts. 1987. Women's perception of the safety of the pill: A survey in eight developing countries. Journal of Biosocial Science 19:313-321.

Fishman, J., J. Schneider, R. J. Herschcopp, and H. L. Bradlow. 1984. Increased estrogen-16α-hydroxylase activity in women with breast and endometrial cancer. Journal of Steroid Biochemistry 20:1077-1081.

Foekens, J. A., H. Portengen, W. L. Van Putten, A. M. A. C. Trapman, J.-C. Reubl, J. Alexia-Figush, and J. G. M. Kiljn. 1989. Prognostic value of receptors for insulin-like growth factor 1, somatostatin, and epidermal growth factor in human breast cancer. Cancer Research 49:7002-7009.

Foote, F. W., and F. E. Stewart. 1941. Lobular carcinoma in situ: A rare form of mammary cancer. American Journal of Pathology 17:491-505.

Fortney, J. A., J. M. Harper, and M. Potts. 1986. Oral contraceptives and life expectancy. Studies in Family Planning 17:117-125.

Frye, R. A., C. C. Beng, and E. T. Liu. 1989. Detection of amplified oncogenes by differential polymerase chain reaction. Oncogene 4:1153-1157.

Garrett, P. A. (Project Manager) and B. S. Hulka (Principal Investigator). Rare HA-RAS alleles and breast cancer. Grant #1-R03-CA52447-01, funded by National Cancer Institute.

Gusterson, B. A., P. Monaghan, R. Mahendran, J. Ellis, and M. J. O'Hare. 1986. Identification of myoepithelial cells in human and rat breasts by anti-common acute lymphoblastic leukemia antigen antibody Al2. Journal of the National Cancer Institute 77:343-347.

Heithoff, K. A., and K. N. Lohr, eds. 1990. Effectiveness and Outcomes in Health Care. Washington, D.C.: National Academy Press.

Hemminki, E., D. L. Kennedy, C. Baum, and S. M. McKinlay. 1988. Prescribing of noncontraceptive estrogens and progestins in the United States, 1974-86. American Journal of Public Health 78:1478-1481.

Huebner, K., A. C. Ferrari, P. Bovi, C. M. Croce, and C. Basilico. 1988. The FGF-related oncogene, K-FGF, maps to human chromosome region 11q13, possibly near int-2. Oncogene Research 3:263-270.

Kay, C. R. 1990. Results from the Royal College of General Practitioners' Oral Contraception Study. Pp. 257-269 in Oral Contraceptives and Breast Cancer, R. D. Mann, ed. Park Ridge, N.J.: The Parthenon Publishing Group.

Kennedy, D. L., C. Baum, and M. B. Forbes. 1985. Noncontraceptive estrogens and progestins: Use patterns over time. Obstetrics and Gynecology 65:441-446.

Kirkland, W. I., H. Yang, T. Jorgensen, C. Langley, and P. Furmanski. 1979. Growth of normal and malignant human mammary epithelial cells in culture. Journal of the National Cancer Institute 63:29-41.

Kramer, W. M., and B. F. Rush. 1973. Mammary duct proliferation in the elderly. Cancer 31:130-137.

Lippman, M. E., and R. B. Dickson. 1989. Mechanisms of growth control in normal and malignant breast epithelium. Recent Progress in Hormone Research 45:383-440.

London, S. J., G. A. Colditz, M. J. Stampfer, W. C. Willett, B. A. Rosner, K. Corsano, and F. E. Speizer. 1990. Lactation and risk of breast cancer in a cohort of US women. American Journal of Epidemiology 132:17-26.

MacMahon, B., P. Cole, T. M. Lin, C. R. Lowe, A. P. Mirra, B. Ravuihar, E. J. Salber, V. G. Valaoras, and S. Yuasa. 1970. Age at first birth and risk of breast cancer. Bulletin of the World Health Organization 43:209.

Mann, R. D., ed. 1990. Oral Contraceptives and Breast Cancer. Park Ridge, N.J.: The Parthenon Publishing Group.

Marchant, D. J., and S. M. Sutton. 1990. Use of mammography—United States, 1990. Morbidity and Mortality Weekly Report 39:621-630.

Mattison, D. R. 1984. How everyday drugs can affect reproduction. Contemporary Obstetrics and Gynecology 24:92-108.

McCarty, K. S., Jr. 1989. Proliferative stimuli in the normal breast: Estrogens or progestins? Human Pathology 20:1137-1138.

McPherson, K. 1990. Summary and update of the Oxford-based studies. Pp. 55-66 in Oral Contraceptives and Breast Cancer, R. D. Mann, ed. Park Ridge, N.J.: The Parthenon Publishing Group.

McTiernan, A., and D. B. Thomas. 1986. Evidence for a protective effect of lactation on risk of breast cancer in young women. American Journal of Epidemiology 124:353-358.

Milburn, M. V., L. Tong, A. M. deVos, A. Brunger, Z. Yamaizumi, S. Nishmura, and S.-H. Kim. 1990. Molecular switch for signal transduction: Structural differences between active and inactive forms of protooncogenic ras proteins. Science 247:939-945.

Mosher, W. D., and W. F. Pratt. 1990. Contraceptive use in the United States, 1973-1988. Advance Data from Vital and Health Statistics, No. 182. Hyattsville, Md.: National Center for Health Statistics.

National Research Council. 1983. Risk Assessment in the Federal Government: Managing the Process. Washington, D.C.: National Academy Press.

National Research Council. 1984. Toxicity Testing: Strategies to Determine Needs and Priorities. Washington, D.C.: National Academy Press.

National Research Council/Institute of Medicine (NRC/IOM). 1990. Developing New Contraceptives: Obstacles and Opportunities, L. Mastroianni, Jr., P. J. Donaldson, and T. T. Kane, eds. Washington, D.C.: National Academy Press.

Osborn, M., and K. Weber. 1983. Biology of disease. Tumor diagnosis by intermediate filament typing: A novel tool for surgical pathology. Laboratory Investigation 48:271-294.

Petersen, O. W., and B. van Deurs. 1988. Growth factor control of myoepithelial-cell differentiation in cultures of human mammary gland. Differentiation 39:197-215.

Resnick, R. M., M. T. E. Conelissen, D. K. Wright, G. H. Eichinger, et al. 1990. Detection and typing of human papillomavirus in archival cervical cancer specimens by DNA amplification with consensus primers. Journal of the National Cancer Institute 82:1477-1484.

Romieu, I., W. C. Willett, G. A. Colditz, M. J. Stampfer, B. Rosner, C. H. Hennekens, and F. E. Speizer. 1990. A prospective study of oral contraceptive use and the risk of breast cancer in women. Pp. 221-243 in Oral Contraceptives and Breast Cancer, R. D. Mann, ed. Park Ridge, N.J.: The Parthenon Publishing Group.

Russo, J., P. Furmanski, and M. A. Rich. 1975. An ultrastructural study of normal human mammary epithelial cells in culture. American Journal of Anatomy 142:221-232.

Smith, H. S., S. R. Wolman, S. H. Dairkee, et al. 1987. Immortalization in culture: Occurrence at a late stage in the progression of breast cancer. Journal of the National Cancer Institute 78:611-615.

Swaneck, G. E., and J. Fishman. 1988. Covalent binding of the endogenous estrogen 16α-hydroxyestrone to estradiol receptor in human breast cancer cells: Characterization and intranuclear localization. Proceedings of the National Academy of Sciences USA 85:7831-7835.

Swift, M., L. L. Kupper, and C. L. Chase. 1990. Effective testing of gene-disease associations. American Journal of Human Genetics 47:266-274.

Taylor-Papadimitriou, J., and E. B. Lane. 1987. Keratin expression in the mammary gland. Pp. 181-215 in The Mammary Gland, M. C. Neville and C. W. Daniel, eds. New York: Plenum Press.

Taylor-Papadimitriou, J., M. Shearer, and R. Tilly. 1977. Some properties of cells cultured from early lactation human milk. Journal of the National Cancer Institute 58:1563-1571.

Thomas, D. B. 1984. Do hormones cause breast cancer? Cancer 53:595-604.

Vessey, M. P. 1990. Results from the Oxford-Family Planning Association Study. Pp. 271-276 in Oral Contraceptives and Breast Cancer, R. D. Mann, ed. Park Ridge, N.J.: The Parthenon Publishing Group.

White, E., C. Y. Lee, and A. R. Kristal. 1990. Evaluation of the increase in breast cancer incidence in relation to mammography use. Journal of the National Cancer Institute 82:1546-1552.

Yuan, J. M., M. C. Yu, R. K. Ross, Y. T. Gao, and B. E. Henderson. 1988. Risk factors for breast cancer in Chinese women in Shanghai. Cancer Research 48:1949-1953.

APPENDIXES

A
Oral Contraceptives and Breast Cancer: A Review of the Epidemiological Evidence with an Emphasis on Younger Women

The possibility of increased breast cancer risk related to oral contraceptive use is a major concern to American women and to the scientific community. Breast cancer incidence in Western countries is relatively high and apparently is increasing. That breast cancer appears to be influenced by other hormonally mediated factors leads to the hypothesis that the high rate of exposure to oral contraceptives among American women may also be associated with this increase.

Examination of cancer incidence data from the Surveillance, Epidemiology, and End Results (SEER) Program of the National Cancer Institute suggests that there has been an overall increase in the incidence of breast cancer, with increases of the largest magnitude occurring among women over age 50 (according to SEER data, approximately 1.2 percent per year since 1974). Age-adjusted incidence rates for breast cancer in women under the age of 50 have also increased since 1973, but the increases have been of a much smaller magnitude—approximately 0.2 percent per year. The use of mammographic screening, which facilitates the detection of cases that might otherwise have gone unnoticed, or at the least detects cases at an earlier point in time, may explain some of this increase, especially in women over age 50. However, because screening recommendations apply

Kathleen E. Malone is a Research Associate at the Fred Hutchinson Cancer Research Center, and a graduate student at the University of Washington, Seattle, Washington.

mainly to middle-aged and older women, screening may not account for much of the increased incidence in young women.

Most of the early research on this topic (i.e., studies conducted prior to 1980) found no association between oral contraceptive use and breast cancer, reassuring many in the research and clinical communities that there was little or no increased risk (Henderson et al., 1974; Sartwell et al., 1977; Ravnihar et al., 1979; Vessey et al., 1979). Investigations reported in the early 1980s offered little to cause observers to change their minds. The majority of studies, including the largest case-control study in the United States, found no consistent suggestion of elevated risk (Kelsey et al., 1981; Vessey et al., 1981, 1982, 1983; Brinton et al., 1982; CASH, 1983; Janerich et al., 1983; Hennekens et al., 1984; Rosenberg et al., 1984; Stadel et al., 1985; Talamini et al., 1985), although several studies reported elevated risk estimates for particular aspects of oral contraceptive use (Paffenbarger et al., 1980; Pike et al., 1981, 1983; Royal College of General Practitioners, 1981; Trapido, 1981; McPherson et al., 1983; Olsson et al., 1985). There was no consistency among these elevated risk estimates.

The picture seems to have changed since 1986. There are a number of studies during this period that do not support an increased risk related to oral contraceptive use, including more analyses of the Cancer and Steroid Hormone (CASH) Study data and the updated analysis of data from the United States nurses' cohort study (CASH, 1986; Ellery et al., 1986; La Vecchia et al., 1986; Lipnick et al., 1986; Romieu et al., 1989; Stanford et al., 1989). But an increasing number of studies have appeared that suggest an elevated risk in relation to some aspects of oral contractive use (Meirik et al., 1986, 1989; Paul et al., 1986; McPherson et al., 1987; Ravnihar et al., 1988; Kay and Hannaford, 1988; Miller et al., 1989; Olsson et al., 1989; U.K. National Case-Control Study Group, 1989). These studies, especially those with positive findings, have received much publicity and generated renewed concern over the safety of oral contraceptives.

CHANGING PROFILE OF ORAL CONTRACEPTIVE USE

Oral contraceptives were introduced in the early 1960s but did not find widespread acceptance until the late 1960s and early 1970s. There are four major types of oral contraceptives. Combination pills, which contain fixed amounts of estrogen and progestin and act by suppressing ovulation, were the first oral contraceptive approved in the United States (in the early 1960s) and have always been the most popular type of pill used. Sequential pills, in which estrogen alone is given for the first two weeks followed by an estrogen-progestin combination during the last six days, were also introduced early but were removed from the U.S. market around 1977 (Piper and Kennedy, 1987). The minipills, or progestin-only pills, introduced in 1972 contain no estrogen and a lower amount of progestin. They do not affect ovulation but rather inhibit ovum transport and implantation by thickening the cervical mucus. They have never had a significant share of the market. Phasic oral contraceptives, combination pills that contain estrogen along with a progestin dose that varies in amount throughout the month, were introduced in 1983 and have since become increasingly popular.

Following the advent of oral contraceptives, two major changes have occurred that must be considered in evaluating the research on oral contraceptives and breast cancer: (1) changes in the formulation of oral contraceptives and (2) changes in the patterns of their use and in the women who use them. Regarding the first change, over the past three decades, the formulations of oral contraceptives have undergone substantial modifications. Both the types and doses of steroids have changed; the doses of both estrogen and progestins have been greatly decreased; several new progestins have entered the market whereas others have been withdrawn; and sequential pills are no longer used. High-estrogen-potency oral contraceptives constituted 94 percent of the United States retail market in 1964, but by 1976 low-estrogen oral contraceptives (less than 50 µg of estrogen), which were introduced in 1967, dominated the market (Piper and Kennedy, 1987). Many of the formulations evaluated in past breast cancer studies are no longer being sold.

The profiles of oral contraceptive users have also changed over time. Oral contraceptives were most commonly used first in the 1960s by married women to space pregnancies and only later by single women as a method to delay a first pregnancy (McPherson and Drife, 1986). Routine prescription to younger single women was not common until the early 1970s in Great Britain and the late 1970s in the United States (McPherson and Drife, 1986). These geographic differences in oral contraceptive prescription patterns have been posited as a possible explanation for some of the differences in study results that have been seen between the two countries. In the United States, only women born since the mid-1940s have had the opportunity to be exposed to long-term use of the pill early in life.

At present the use of oral contraceptives is an extremely prevalent exposure among young women. With the recent epidemic of teenage pregnancies in the United States, routine prescription to teenage girls as young as age 13 is not uncommon. Unpublished data from a case-control study conducted by the author and colleagues of breast cancer diagnosed between 1983 and 1988 in young women born after 1944 in Seattle, Washington, showed that 92 percent of both the cases and controls reported "ever" having used oral contraceptives; among women under age 20 the proportion of "ever" use increased to 100 percent.

BIOLOGICAL PLAUSIBILITY

An important criterion for evaluating causality is the biological plausibility of the relationship. Estrogen causes proliferation of breast tissue and would be expected to increase breast cancer risk by stimulating growth of stem cells and intermediate cells (Thomas, 1984). Progestin causes alveolar cell growth in the estrogen-primed breast, but it also causes differentiation. It is unclear, therefore, whether the predicted net effect would be to increase or decrease breast cancer risk.

The influence of estrogen and progestin on breast epithelium proliferation and differentiation appears to differ with age. Cancer risk is thought to be a function of the number of cells at risk, which varies with age. It is possible to posit that any carcinogenic risk of oral contraceptives may be strongly mediated by age of exposure or by the timing of exposure in relation to other events that are thought to affect epithelial proliferation or differentiation (e.g., menarche, first full-term pregnancy).

The etiology of breast cancer has strong hormonal themes: oophorectomy decreases risk, early menarche and late menopause increase risk, late age at first full-term pregnancy increases risk. These effects seem to last for decades. Thus, if use early in life affects risk, it may be many years before deleterious outcomes are seen. It is possible that the studies conducted thus far have not allowed an adequate interval between exposure to oral contraceptives and the onset of breast cancer, so that even if an association were present, it might not yet be detectable. Thus, vigilance must be maintained and investigation of this issue should continue in the future—even though we might conclude, based on current data, that findings are too inconsistent to be alarming at present.

EPIDEMIOLOGICAL STUDIES OF BREAST CANCER
AND ORAL CONTRACEPTIVES

As mentioned earlier, the studies conducted prior to 1980 carry little suggestion of an increased risk for breast cancer in relation to oral contraceptive use. These studies focused on cases diagnosed before 1975; therefore, they included a large proportion of women who, because of their birth years, had little opportunity to have ever used oral contraceptives or to have used oral contraceptives for a long time, and virtually no opportunity for exposure at an early age. For these reasons, as well as the briefness of the time between exposure and diagnosis, studies conducted before 1980 cannot contribute any insight into the current controversy and are largely ignored in this review. Unfortunately, these same difficulties plague some of the studies published in the early 1980s as well. Therefore, although studies from the early 1980s are included in this review, the emphasis is on more recent research.

"Ever" Use of Oral Contraceptives

Table A-1 presents a summary of the findings related to "ever" use of oral contraceptives and risk of breast cancer. Twenty-five of the 30 studies for which a relative risk for "ever" use was reported had relative risks (RR) close to 1.0. Two of the five studies that report elevated risk estimates for "ever" use of the pill are ones for which questions with regard either to basic study design, low response rates, or low exposure prevalence have been raised (Olsson et al., 1989; Miller et al., 1989). Overall, there is no evidence of increased risk of breast cancer in women who meet the criterion of "ever" using oral contraceptives. The finding of no association between "ever" use of oral contraceptives and breast cancer risk has been quite consistent throughout the past 20 years of research.

"Ever" use of oral contraceptives is probably too crude a measure to provide much insight into any relationship with breast cancer risk because such use is so common an exposure that it typically encompasses more than 90 percent of all young women. Further, interpretation is difficult because there are subgroups of women who try oral contraceptives but stop—because of side effects—soon after they start. Women who never use oral contraceptives may be a unique subgroup. For instance, they may have an increased family history of breast cancer, health problems that contraindicate the use of oral contraceptives, or an increased awareness or suspicion of undiagnosed infertility; these factors, in turn, may relate to both their decision not to use oral contraceptives and their risk for breast cancer.

Duration of Oral Contraceptive Use

There was little suggestion of increased risk related to long-term use of oral contraceptives in any of the studies published prior to 1986. Of the case-control studies published since that time, seven

TABLE A-1 Summary of Risk Estimates for "Ever" Use of Oral
Contraceptives

Author/Year	Relative Risk[a]	Confidence Interval
Paffenbarger et al., 1980		
Premenopausal	1.1[b]	
Postmenopausal	1.2[b]	
Pike et al., 1981	1.2	0.7-1.9
Royal College of General		
Practitioners, 1981 (cohort)	1.2	0.8-1.7
Trapido, 1981 (cohort)	0.8	0.7-1.2
Vessey et al., 1981 (cohort)	1.0	0.6-1.6
Brinton et al., 1982	1.1	0.8-1.4
Harris et al., 1982	0.8	0.6-1.3
Vessey et al., 1982	0.9	0.7-1.2
Vessey et al., 1983	1.0	0.8-1.2
Hennekens et al., 1984	1.0	0.9-1.2
Rosenberg et al., 1984	1.0	0.9-1.2
Stadel et al., 1985 (CASH[d])	1.0	0.9-1.2
Talamini et al., 1985	0.7	0.4-1.4
CASH,[d] 1986	1.0	0.9-1.1
Ellery et al., 1986	0.9	0.6-1.5
LaVecchia et al., 1986	1.1	0.8-1.5
Lipnick et al., 1986	1.0	0.8-1.3
Meirik et al., 1986	1.4	1.1-1.9
Miller et al., 1986	0.9	0.7-1.4
Paul et al., 1986	0.9	0.7-1.3
Lee et al., 1987	1.2	0.8-1.8
McPherson et al., 1987	1.2	0.8-1.6
Kay and Hannaford, 1988 (cohort)		
Age at diagnosis		
25-29	2.5	1.0-52.5
30-34	3.3	1.3-8.8
< 35	2.4	1.0-5.8
35-39	0.9	0.3-3.2
0-44	1.0	0.9-1.1
45-49	1.8	0.8-4.2
50-54	1.8	0.2-20.3
All ages	1.2	0.9-1.6
Schlesselman et al., 1988 (CASH[d])	0.9	0.8-1.0
Ravnihar et al., 1988	1.6	1.3-2.1
Yuan et al., 1988	1.1	0.7-1.5
Miller et al., 1989	2.0	1.4-2.9
Olsson et al., 1989	1.8[c]	
Romieu et al., 1989 (cohort)	1.1	1.0-1.2
Stanford et al., 1989	1.0	0.9-1.2
WHO,[d] 1990	1.2	1.0-1.3

[a]Reference group = "never" users.
[b]Confidence intervals not provided by author.
[c]Crude relative risk calculated from data provided in paper.
[d]WHO = World Health Organization; CASH = Cancer and Steroid Hormone Study.

reported an excess risk for use of long duration. Table A-2 presents a summary of reported risk estimates for long-term use. The largest case-control study of breast cancer conducted to date, the CASH study, showed no evidence of an association of breast cancer risk and long-term use of oral contraceptives among women aged 20 to 54 (CASH, 1986). Yet despite its size (the study comprised more that 4,700 cases and a similar number of controls in eight geographic regions of the United States) the majority of the women were over age 45. Coupled with the early diagnosis years (1980-1982), it is possible that this study was conducted too early to detect any association between oral contraceptives and breast cancer. The major reproductive years for most of these women occurred before the height of popularity of the pill. A number of the other studies among women up to the age of 65 have also found no pattern related to long durations of use, suggesting no increase in risk related to long-term oral contraceptive use in the aggregate or perhaps no increase in risk with long-term use that does not begin at an early age (Ellery et al., 1986; La Vecchia et al., 1986; Paul et al., 1986; Stanford et al., 1989). A Yugoslavian study of women under age 55, however, found an RR of 2.4 for oral contraceptive use exceeding seven years, as well as a significant dose-response pattern (Ravnihar et al., 1988). Recently, the World Health Organization (WHO) study, a multinational case-control study conducted in three developed and seven developing countries, reported a suggestive dose-response pattern of increasing risk with years of oral contraceptive use (WHO, 1990); this association, however, could well be attributable to a recency effect since risk was highest in current users and steadily declined with time since last exposure.

In recent years, a large number of studies have focused on breast cancer risk in women under age 45. Meirik and colleagues (1986) published the first report suggesting a dose-response relationship with duration of oral contraceptive use among young women: for use of 8 to 11 years, an RR of 1.4 was found; for 12 or more years of use, a 2.2-fold excess risk of breast cancer was found. Paul and colleagues (1986) reported an RR of 4.6 for use of 10 or more years among women aged 25-34. McPherson and coworkers (1987) found an increased RR of 1.8 for use exceeding 11 years among a group of British women through age 45. The fact that U.K. prescription patterns were about five years ahead of those in the United States has been offered as a possible explanation for the earlier emergence of positive studies from the United Kingdom.

A hospital-based case-control study conducted in the northeastern United States (Miller et al., 1989) among women under age 45 ob-

TABLE A-2 Summary of Risk Estimates for Lifetime Duration of Oral Contraceptive Use

Author/Year	Age	Diagnosis Dates	Duration of Use (years)	Relative Risk[a]	Confidence Interval
Vessey et al., 1983	16-50	1968-80	≤1	0.9	0.7-1.1
			>1-4	1.0	0.8-1.3
			>4-8	1.2	0.8-1.6
			>8	1.0	0.7-1.5
Hennekens et al., 1984	30-55	1960-76	<1	1.1	0.9-1.4
			1-2	1.1	0.9-1.5
			3-4	0.7	0.5-1.1
			5-9	1.1	0.8-1.4
			10+	0.7	0.4-1.3
Rosenberg et al., 1984	20-59	1976-81	<1	0.9	0.7-1.1
			1-4	0.9	0.8-1.2
			5-9	1.3	1.0-1.7
			10+	0.8	0.5-1.3
CASH,[b] 1986	20-54	1980-82	6-9	1.0[c]	
			10-14	1.1	
			15+	0.6	
Ellery et al., 1986	25-64	1980-82	2.1-6	0.7	0.3-1.5
			6+	1.0	0.5-2.0
La Vecchia et al., 1986	<60	1982-85	<2	1.0	0.7-1.4
			>2	1.1	0.7-1.6
Lipnick et al., 1986	30-55 in 1976	1976-80	<1	0.9	0.7-1.3
			1-2	0.8	0.6-1.1
			3-4	1.0	0.7-1.4
			5-9	1.2	0.8-1.5
			10+	1.3	0.9-1.9
Meirik et al., 1986	<45	1984-85	4-7	1.2	0.8-1.9
			8-11	1.4	0.8-2.3
			12+	2.2	1.2-4.0
Paul et al., 1986	25-54	1983-85	6-9	0.8[c]	
			10+	1.0	
Lee et al., 1987	25-58	1982-84	5-9	1.2	0.6-2.3
			10+	1.0	0.4-2.6
McPherson et al., 1987	16-64	1980-84			
Among women	<45		4-12	1.2	0.8-1.8
			13+	1.8	0.8-3.9
Among women	45+		4-12	1.1	0.7-1.6
			13+	0.8	0.4-1.8
Kay and Hannaford, 1988 (cohort)	15-45 in 1968-69				
Among ages	30-34		4-5	4.1	1.1-14.5
			6-7	2.2	0.4-11.8
			8-9	2.5	0.3-22.4
			10+	10.2	1.1-91.0
Ravnihar et al., 1988	25-54	1980-83	4-7	1.7	1.2-2.5
			8+	2.4	1.5-2.8

TABLE A-2 (Continued)

Author/Year	Age	Diagnosis Dates	Duration of Use (years)	Relative Risk[a]	Confidence Interval
Stadel et al., 1988	20-54	1980-82	8-11[d]		
	20-44				
			Menarche <13	2.7	1.2-6.3
			Menarche 13+	0.9	0.5-2.1
	45-54				
			Menarche <13	0.4	0.1-2.2
			Menarche 13+	0.8	0.2-3.1
Jick et al., 1989	<43	1975-83	10+	1.4	0.4-4.6
Miller et al., 1989	25-44	1983-86	5-9	1.9	1.1-3.3
			10+	4.1	1.8-9.3
Romieu et al., 1989	30-55	1976-86	5-<10	1.1	1.0-1.4
(cohort)	in 1976		10-<14	1.1	0.8-1.4
			15+	1.1	0.5-2.4
Stanford et al., 1989	Older	1973-80	<1	0.9	0.7-1.2
			2-4	0.8	0.6-1.1
			5-9	1.2	0.9-1.6
			10-14	1.0	0.7-1.5
			15+	0.7	0.3-1.6
U.K. National Case-Control Study Group, 1989	<36	1982-85	4-8	1.4	1.0-2.1
			>8	1.7	1.2-2.6
			Parous women 4-8	1.4[c]	
			>8	1.6	
			Nulliparous women 4-8	1.4	
			>8	2.3	
WHO,[b] 1990	<63	1979-86	<1	1.1	1.0-1.3
			1-2	1.0	0.8-1.2
			3-8	1.2	1.0-1.4
			>8	1.6	1.2-2.0

[a]Reference group = "never" users.
[b]WHO = World Health Organization; CASH = Cancer and Steroid Hormone Study.
[c]Confidence intervals not provided by author.
[d]Years of use among nulliparous women only.

served a twofold excess risk for oral contraceptive use of five to nine years' duration and a fourfold excess risk for use of 10 or more years. Questions have been raised about Miller's findings because of concern about the appropriateness of the hospitalized control group and because there appears to be a lower proportion of exposed controls than would be expected from national data. A well-conducted study in the United Kingdom (U.K. National Case-Control Study Group, 1989) among women under age 36 recently reported a significant dose-response pattern for duration of use. Oral contraceptive use of 49 to 96 months was associated with a 1.4-fold excess risk, and use exceeding 96 months was associated with a 1.7-fold excess breast cancer risk. This case-control study was one of the few that was able to validate the self-reported data on oral contraceptive use so as to rule out the often-raised criticism of recall bias.

Conflicting observations have been recorded among the three large prospective cohort studies. The largest, the Nurses Health study in the United States (Romieu et al., 1989), found no increase in risk for any duration of use (or for any other aspect of oral contraceptive use except current use). Current use of oral contraceptives was associated with an overall adjusted RR of 1.5. This excess risk was confined to women between ages 40 and 50. Tumors in current users were reported to be larger and to have more lymph node involvement at the time of diagnosis than were tumors in women not currently using oral contraceptives. The Oxford cohort in the United Kingdom has seen no evidence of increased risk related to oral contraceptive use (Vessey et al., 1989). However, the Royal College of General Practitioners cohort in the United Kingdom reported excess breast cancer risk for longer durations of oral contraceptive use, although there was no consistent dose-response pattern (Kay and Hannaford, 1988). In this cohort, there were inconsistent, mildly elevated risks for duration of use among women of all ages. In two subgroups, women ages 30 to 34 and women who were parity 1, much higher risks were seen—as high as a 10-fold excess risk for use of 10 or more years. Both of the cohorts formed in the United Kingdom began recruitment in 1968 and excluded women not involved in a married or living as married relationship (Kay and Hannaford, 1988; Vessey et al., 1989). The Nurses' Health study recruited women aged 30-55 in 1976 (Romieu et al., 1989). All three of these cohorts may have been initiated too early to include many women born recently enough to have had the opportunity to use oral contraceptives at a young age or for a long duration.

Oral Contraceptive Use Before First Full-term Pregnancy or Before Age 25

It is possible that oral contraceptives may be especially influential at or in relation to particular reproductive milestones. Because of the increasing frequency of use of the pill at young ages, and because of the possibility of increased susceptibility of breast tissue to hormonal exposures during young ages when breast development is still ongoing and when endogenous hormone concentrations are still increasing, there has been mounting interest in the evaluation of breast cancer risk in relation to use at young ages. Findings regarding any relationship between use of oral contraceptives before the first full-term pregnancy (FFTP) or before age 25 have been inconsistent. A factor that further complicates the picture is that some investigators report on use before FFTP only among parous women, some consider parous and nulliparous women combined, and others investigate only nulliparous women. Table A-3 summarizes the findings regarding oral contraceptive use before FFTP.

The vast majority of investigations of the relationship between oral contraceptive use prior to FFTP and breast cancer risk have focused on women under age 45. Pike's 1981 study was the first to report an adverse effect from oral contraceptive use prior to FFTP, observing an RR of 2.3 for five to eight years of oral contraceptive use preceding FFTP and an RR of 3.5 for more than eight years use before FFTP. One limitation of this study, however, was a low response rate for the cases. A threefold excess risk was reported by McPherson and colleagues (1983) for use exceeding four years' duration before FFTP and was accompanied by the suggestion of a dose-response relationship. The McPherson team's 1987 report observed a twofold excess risk of breast cancer for one to four years of use before FFTP and a 2.6-fold excess risk for use exceeding four years' duration prior to FFTP among nulliparous and parous women combined. Meirik and coworkers' (1986, 1989) reports on Swedish and Norwegian women revealed an increased risk for eight or more years of use before FFTP in the aggregate as well as in both nulliparous and parous women when examined separately (all women: RR = 2.0, confidence interval (CI) = 1.8-4.2; nulliparous women: RR = 4.3, CI = 1.4-13.1; parous women: RR = 1.7, CI = 0.7-4.2). There is some suggestion in Meirik's data that use before FFTP may be related to overall long duration of oral contraceptive exposure. This may well be true for some of the other studies but was not addressed in the tables or text of most other papers.

Two recent studies also observed increased risks for oral contraceptive use prior to FFTP, although both studies have been criticized because of possible design limitations. The hospital-based study by Miller and colleagues (1989), for which possible limitations were mentioned previously, found a 1.6-fold excess risk of breast cancer for oral contraceptive use preceding FFTP that exceeded four years. In the Swedish study by Olsson and coworkers (1989), an RR of 1.8 (CI = 1.0-3.2) was observed for three or fewer years of oral contraceptive

TABLE A-3   Summary of Risk Estimates for Oral Contraceptive Use Before First Full-term Pregnancy

Author/Year	Age	Diagnosis Dates	Duration of Use (Years)	Relative Risk	Confidence Interval
McPherson et al., 1983	<45	1980-83	<1	1.2	0.5-2.8
			1.1-4	1.7	0.8-3.8
			>4	3.1	1.3-7.5
Stadel et al., 1985[a]	20-54	1980-82	1.1-4	1.1	0.9-1.5
			>4	1.2	0.9-1.6
Meirik et al., 1986	<45	1984-85	4-7	1.0	0.6-1.7
			8+	2.0	1.8-4.2
Miller et al., 1986	<45	1977-83	3-4	0.8	0.4-1.6
			5-6	1.5	0.6-4.0
			7+	1.4	0.6-3.2
Paul et al., 1986	25-54	1983-85	<2	0.9	
			2-3	0.8	
			4-5	0.7	
			6+	0.6	
McPherson et al., 1987[a]	16-64	1980-84	1.1-4	2.0	1.0-3.8
			>4	2.6	1.3-5.4
Stadel, 1988[c]	20-54	1980-82	4-7	1.3	0.7-2.6
			8-11	2.7	1.2-6.3
			12+	11.8	1.4-95.7
Jick et al., 1989	<43	1978-83	4+	1.3	0.3-4.6
Meirik et al., 1986	<45	1984-85			
Among nulliparous			<4	2.8	1.1-7.4
women			4-7	1.0	0.3-3.3
			8+	4.3	1.4-13.1
Among parous			<4	1.2	0.8-1.8
women			4-7	1.2	0.7-2.2
			8+	1.7	0.7-4.2
Miller et al., 1989	25-44	1983-86			
Among nulliparous			1-4	1.0	0.4-2.7
women			5+	1.6	0.7-3.6
Among parous			1-4	2.5	1.2-5.2
women			5+	1.3	0.4-4.0
Olsson et al., 1989	<46	1979-80	0-3	1.8	1.0-3.2
		and	4-7	1.7	1.1-3.8
		1982-85	8+	2.1	0.8-4.7
Romieu et al., 1989[d]	30-55	1976-86	<1	1.0	0.7-1.4
	in 1976		1-<3	1.1	0.8-1.6
			3+	0.8	0.4-1.7
WHO,[e] 1990	<63	1979-86	<2	0.8	0.6-1.1
			2+	1.2	0.8-2.0
			Ever	0.9	0.7-1.2

[a]Data are for women younger than 45 years of age.
[b]Confidence intervals not provided by author.
[c]Results are for nulliparous women aged 20-44 whose menarche occurred before age 13.
[d]Results are for parous premenopausal women.
[e]WHO = World Health Organization.

use prior to FFTP, an RR of 1.7 (CI = 1.1-3.8) for four to seven years of use before FFTP, and an RR of 2.1 (CI = 0.8-4.7) for use of eight or more years before FFTP. Different interviewers were used for cases versus controls, however, and the response rates were rather low in this study, raising concerns about the findings.

A number of analyses found no suggestion of increased breast cancer risk for oral contraceptive use before FFTP (Paul et al., 1986; Jick et al., 1989; Romieu et al., 1989; WHO, 1990). Overall consideration of oral contraceptive use before FFTP in the complete Cancer and Steroid Hormone study data revealed no suggestion of excess breast cancer risk in the study's first report on the entire data set (Stadel et al., 1985). However, in a recent analysis of a "high-risk" subgroup of the CASH study subjects—nulliparous women with an early age of menarche diagnosed with breast cancer before age 45— an excess risk of breast cancer was seen in relation to increasing duration of oral contraceptive use (Stadel et al., 1988). The risk for oral contraceptive use of 8 to 11 years was 2.7, and the risk for use of 12 or more years was 11.8. A recent letter by Peto (1989) presented a crude reanalysis of the published CASH data that challenged an earlier conclusion of the study of no excess risk for use before FFTP.

Eight studies, which are summarized in Table A-4, have reported on use before age 25. Three studies (Stadel et al., 1985; Miller et al., 1986; McPherson et al., 1987) have shown no indication of a relationship with breast cancer risk, whereas four (Pike et al., 1983; Meirik et al., 1986; Olsson et al., 1989; WHO, 1990) suggest a positive relationship and one (Paul et al., 1986) suggests a protective effect. Pike and coworkers' 1983 study, in an expansion of the 1981 investigation, observed a significant dose-response pattern of increased risk for increased duration of use before age 25. For such use exceeding five years' duration, there was a 4.9-fold excess risk. In the data from Meirik and colleagues (1986), among Swedish and Norwegian women, there was no elevation in risk for use of less than eight years' duration prior to age 25, but there was an increased risk of 2.7 (CI = 0.7-11.0) for use of eight years or more before age 25. The Olsson team's 1989 study, also among Swedish women, reported a suggestive dose-response pattern for increasing duration of oral contraceptive use prior to age 25, with a 1.6-fold excess risk for use of less than three years before age 25, a twofold excess risk for use of three to five years, and a 5.3-fold excess risk for use exceeding five years.

A major challenge in interpreting many of the studies of use at a young age lies in separating the effects related to use early in life from effects associated with longer durations of exposure. More attention needs to be given to this issue in future analyses, particularly in populations in which the majority of the women were born recently.

TABLE A-4   Summary of Risk Estimates for Oral Contraceptive Use Before Age 25

Author/Year[a]	Duration of Use (years)	Relative Risk	Confidence Interval
Pike et al., 1983	Ever	1.6	1.1-2.3
	<3	1.3	0.8-2.0
	3-4	1.7	1.0-2.7
	5-6	2.0	1.1-3.6
	>6	4.9	1.9-13.4
Stadel et al., 1985	<=2	1.2	0.8-1.9
High-progestogen-	2-3	1.3	0.8-2.1
potency use	4-11	1.1	0.6-1.9
	12+	1.3	0.5-3.3
Meirik et al., 1986	<4	1.1	0.8-1.5
	4-7	1.1	0.7-1.8
	8+	2.7	0.7-11.0
Miller et al., 1986	Ever	1.0	0.7-1.6
	<1	0.8	0.4-1.5
	1-2	1.0	0.6-1.6
	3-4	1.3	0.7-2.3
	5+	1.1	0.4-2.9
Paul et al., 1986	<2	1.2[b]	
	2-3	1.0	
	4-5	0.7	
	6+	0.6	
Olsson et al., 1989	0-2	1.6	0.9-2.8
	3-5	2.0	1.1-3.5
	>5	5.3	2.1-13.2
WHO,[c] 1990	<1	1.0	0.8-1.3
	1-<2	0.8	0.6-1.1
	2-<3	1.5	1.0-2.3
	≥ =3	1.5	1.0-2.3

[a]The table does not include data from McPherson et al. (1987) because the report of the study did not provide risk estimates. The proportions reported, however, suggest no increase in risk by duration of oral contraceptive use before age 25.
[b]Confidence intervals not provided by author.
[c]WHO = World Health Organization.

Duration Since First Use of Oral Contraceptives (Latency)

It has been suggested that long-term latent effects that have been missed might be the alternative explanation for many of the studies with negative findings.   More than 10 studies have presented such analyses with no demonstration of a consistent latency pattern (Brinton et al., 1982; Harris et al., 1982; Vessey et al., 1983; Rosenberg et al.,

1984; Ellery et al., 1986; Meirik et al., 1986; La Vecchia et al., 1986; Paul et al., 1986; Lee et al., 1987; Ravnihar et al., 1988; Schlesselman et al., 1988). It is possible, however, that these studies were conducted too early to see such an effect.

Use of Oral Contraceptives in High-Risk Subgroups

Although many investigators adjust for high-risk factors (e.g., family history of breast cancer, history of benign breast disease) in their analyses, only a subset have examined oral contraceptive use within each of these strata. Furthermore, of the few studies that have examined oral contraceptive use in each strata, the majority have limited their definition of use to "ever/never" and their definition of the high-risk subgroups to fairly crude delineations (i.e., "ever/never" had sister with breast cancer). These approaches are unfortunate because they may well miss important modifying relationships that cannot be detected at such a crude level.

With regard to family history of breast cancer, the bulk of the studies have detected no substantial differences in the risk related to oral contraceptive use for women with and without this factor (Miller et al., 1989; Murray et al., 1989; Romieu et al., 1989). Brinton and colleagues (1982) found no differences in women with and without a mother with breast cancer but did see differences in women with and without a sister with breast cancer.

Elevated risks have been observed for oral contraceptive use among women with a history of benign breast disease (Fasal and Paffenbarger, 1975; Lees et al., 1978; Brinton et al., 1982; Janerich et al., 1983); but more work is needed to evaluate specific histologic types of benign breast disease in terms of both breast cancer risk and relationship to use of the pill. Some past analyses failed to distinguish between oral contraceptive use before and after the diagnosis of benign breast disease (Stadel and Schlesselman, 1986). In addition, not much has been done to examine histologic subgroups of breast cancer for the possibility of differential relationships with oral contraceptive exposure.

Steroidal Potency of Various Formulations

The hormonal contents of oral contraceptives have been examined by a number of classification schemes related to potency, brand, and type of estrogen (Brinton et al., 1982; Harris et al., 1982; Pike et al., 1983; Vessey et al., 1983; Stadel et al., 1985; Ellery et al., 1986; CASH, 1986; Miller et al., 1986; McPherson et al., 1987; Schlesselman et al.,

1987; Ravnihar et al., 1988). Not one of these approaches, however, has consistently exhibited a relationship with breast cancer risk.

ISSUES TO CONSIDER IN REVIEWING
THE EPIDEMIOLOGICAL EVIDENCE

In attempting to evaluate the accumulated research, several issues should be considered. First, the design and conduct of each study should be examined to detect possible limitations that could have affected the results. Specific factors such as the fundamental design (case-control or follow-up study) and the proportion of eligible subjects who participated in the study, or in a follow-up design, are salient to interpretation of the findings. Several of the previously mentioned studies suffered from low response rates or large losses to follow-up (Janerich et al., 1983; Kay and Hannaford, 1988). If these losses are great, the validity of the case-control study is compromised because of the possibility of differential exposure distributions in the responders versus the nonresponders. In a follow-up study, similar questions arise concerning the possible differential distribution of disease occurrence. Table A-5 itemizes the following characteristics for most of the studies addressed here: diagnosis dates and the ages of women at the time of diagnosis, proportion of cases and controls who participated, sample size, proportion of cases and controls who reported "ever" using oral contraceptives, and whether controls were secured from hospitals.

TABLE A-5 Summary of Characteristics of Case-Control and Cohort Studies of the Relationship of Oral Contraceptive Use and Breast Cancer Risk

Author/Year	Diagnosis Dates	Ages	Response Rates (Percentage) of Cases (Controls)	Number of Cases	Percentage of Cases (Controls) Using Oral Contraceptives
Case-Control Studies					
Rosenberg et al., 1984[a]	1976-81	<60	n.a. n.a.	1,191	33 (33)
CASH, 1986	1980-82	<55	80 (83)	4,711	60 (62)
Ellery et al., 1986[a]	1980-82	<65	n.a. n.a.	141	48 (42)
LaVecchia et al., 1986[a]	1982-85	<60	n.a. n.a.	776	13 (14)

TABLE A-5 (Continued)

Author/Year	Diagnosis Dates	Ages	Response Rates (Percentage) of Cases (Controls)	Number of Cases	Percentage of Cases (Controls) Using Oral Contraceptives
Miller et al., 1986[a]	1977-83	<45	96? 96?	521	60 (59)
Paul et al., 1986	1983-85	<55	79 (81)	433	72 (79)
Lee et al., 1987	1982-84	<59	67 (93)	171	34 (43)
McPherson et al., 1987[a]	1980-84	<65	n.a. n.a.	1,125	38 (39)
Ravnihar et al., 1988[a]	1980-83	<55	n.a. n.a.	534	30 (30)
Yuan et al., 1988	1984-85	<70	94 (99)	534	18 (18)
Jick et al., 1989[a]	1975-83	<43	70 (69)	127	61 (71)
Meirik et al., 1989, 1986	1984-85	<45	88 (85)	422	77 (78)
Miller et al., 1989[a]	1983-86	<45	96	407	72 (59)
Olsson et al., 1989	1979-85	<46	n.a. (92)	174	82 (72)
Stanford et al., 1989 (screening program)	1973-80	<82	78 (83)	2,022	24 (24)
U.K. National Case-Control Study Group, 1989	1982-85	<36	72 (89)	755	91 (89)
WHO, 1990[a]	1979-86	<63	94.2 (94.6)	2,116	34 (34)
Cohort Studies					
Kay and Hannaford, 1988[c]	1968-85	28.8[d]		239	60
Romieu et al., 1989[a]	1976-86	30-55 in 1976		1,799	48
Vessey et al., 1989[b]	1968-87	25-39 in 1968	n.a.	189	52

NOTE: WHO = World Health Organization; n.a. = not available; CASH = Cancer and Steroid Hormone Study.

[a]Controls were recruited from hospitals.
[b]The study dropped women who had ever used oral contraceptives but whose use was less than 8 years in duration.
[c]Of the original cohort, 61.7 percent were lost to follow-up.
[d]Mean age in 1968.

The sample size of a study must be large enough to allow the detection of an effect or to rule out with a certain amount of confidence the presence of an effect. A number of past studies (i.e., Kelsey et al., 1978; Harris et al., 1982; Olsson et al., 1985; Ellery et al., 1986; Lee et al., 1987; Jick et al., 1989) may not have had adequate power to evaluate the relationship of oral contraceptives and breast cancer. In addition, sample sizes need to be even larger to examine the interrelationships of other risk factors with oral contraceptive use (Greenland, 1983; Smith and Day, 1984).

In a case-control study, the method of ascertaining cases and controls should be carefully considered, as well as the degree to which the controls represent the population from which the cases were drawn. Concern has been raised about the validity of conducting studies in hospital settings, especially referral or tertiary care hospitals, because it is virtually impossible to identify the population from which the cases arose. The usual approach for selecting controls is to recruit them from among the other patients in the same hospital who are seeking care for other diseases. The difficulty lies in deciding what conditions these patients can and cannot have in order to be an appropriate comparison group. Any condition known to be associated with the exposure or with the disease should be excluded. As the number of exclusions increases, questions arise as to the select nature of the control group; unfortunately, it is impossible to be sure of the direction of the bias that might result from such selectivity. One could hypothesize that the controls with these other medical conditions that have led to hospitalization are less likely to be oral contraceptive users; in that case, however, the controls would produce an underestimate of the population's use of the pill, and the observed risks would be spuriously high. Quite a few of the reviewed studies were conducted in hospital settings (Paffenbarger et al., 1980; Kelsey et al., 1981; Vessey et al., 1982, 1983; McPherson et al., 1983, 1987; Rosenberg et al., 1984; Talamini et al., 1985; Ellery et al., 1986; La Vecchia et al., 1986; Miller et al., 1986, 1989; Ravnihar et al., 1988).

Most recently, the study by Miller and colleagues (1989) was criticized because of its low proportion of pill-exposed controls; the proportion exposed was lower than that observed in national survey data for women in the age group studied. This result raises questions about bias in the selection of the hospital controls (Spirtas, 1989).

A second issue involves any bias that might arise in the ascertainment of exposure. All of the case-control studies reviewed here relied on interview data, although one—the U.K. National Case-Control Study Group (1989)—was able to review medical records to evaluate recall.

Another study (Olsson et al., 1989) violated a basic design principle by having a different interviewer for cases and controls. Third, it is necessary to understand and incorporate into analyses (when appropriate) the other important breast cancer risk factors, such as age of first full-term pregnancy, number of live births, age of menarche, family history of breast cancer, and history of benign breast disease. Some of these risk factors, as well as some other factors, may also affect the decision to use oral contraceptives, the age of first and last use, and the lifetime duration of use. These and other factors may modify or be modified by the relationship of oral contraceptives to breast cancer risk.

Fourth, whether the women in a study had the opportunity to be exposed to oral contraceptives deserves attention. The most obvious example of this issue is when a study includes a large number of women who were born early enough that oral contraceptives were not even on the market during their prime reproductive years. All of the studies before 1980 as well as a number of the studies in the early 1980s were constrained in this way. Extreme examples include La Vecchia and colleagues (1986), with only 14 percent of the study subjects having ever used oral contraceptives; Stanford and coworkers (1989), with 24 percent having used them; and Lee and colleagues (1987), with 41 percent having used them.

When birth year and opportunity for exposure to oral contraceptives are examined in the context of the possible latency period for breast cancer, it becomes apparent that many of the already completed studies may have been unable to evaluate the relationship of oral contraceptives and breast cancer, especially in regard to use at younger ages as well as premenopausal disease onset. For example, the studies of radiation effects on breast cancer suggest a latency interval of at least 15 years, which must be factored into efforts to detect an expected association. Presuming oral contraceptives have a promotion-al effect, the time interval until a detectable lesion is present is unknown. Studies that include women diagnosed before a certain point in time may not have allowed an adequate interval between exposure to oral contraceptives and onset of breast cancer. In this instance, even if an association were present, it might not be detectable in these women.

More subtle examples related to exposure opportunity that need consideration in future analyses include sterilization, hysterectomy, and infertility, all of which necessarily affect the need and timing for any method of contraception.

DISCUSSION

The one conclusive statement that can be made concerning the sum of the epidemiological evidence of a relationship between oral contraceptives and breast cancer is that there has been a remarkable lack of consistency in the findings. However, an increasing number of the recent studies suggest that there are subgroups of women who may be at increased risk of breast cancer owing to their pattern of oral contraceptive use. Of these groups, the one of most concern may be those women with long-term use beginning at a young age. The findings for use before the first full-term pregnancy or before age 25, or just for overall long duration of use are certainly suggestive and do not permit the conclusion that there is no relationship between use of the pill and breast cancer risk. Use of oral contraceptives at a young age has increased over the past 20 years, and the possible risk of breast cancer associated with early use is an important public health issue. Why would we only now be seeing an increased risk for long-term use at a young age? There are several possible explanations:

1. Women who use oral contraceptives are required to visit their health care provider on a regular basis to secure a renewal of their prescription. Thus, it is possible that oral contraceptive users are seen by the health care system more frequently than other women, and may receive more frequent medical surveillance, including breast exams and even mammograms. This hypothesis has led to the suggestion that women with breast cancer who use oral contraceptives are detected and diagnosed earlier than nonusers. Little is known about the natural progression of breast lesions; thus, the detection of breast cancer through mammography may indeed pick up some cases of breast cancer that might have otherwise gone undetected for many years. (This may be especially true of in situ breast cancers.) Several recent studies have incorporated into their analyses a consideration of such factors as the stage of disease, the frequency of breast self-exams and physician exams, and the frequency of mammograms as a way to account for the impact of increased surveillance (McPherson et al., 1987; Kay and Hannaford, 1988; U.K. National Case-Control Study Group, 1989). Because oral contraceptives have always required prescriptions, it seems unlikely that detection bias could be contributing enough new noise to the analyses of breast cancer and oral contraceptives to account completely for the emergence of these recent positive findings.

2. In recent years, the controversy about the relationship between oral contraceptive use and breast cancer risk has received much atten-

tion in the lay press. Unfortunately, there are indications that positive studies receive greater publicity than negative studies. Recent studies therefore have been conducted in an environment in which many participants are familiar with the hypothesis of interest. Many epidemiological studies rely heavily on a woman's memory to ascertain details of pill use; consequently, the issue of recall bias has been raised as a possible explanation for some of the positive studies. The specific scenario of concern is one in which women with breast cancer, because of their diagnosis, ruminate about possible causes and dwell heavily on an exposure that they believe may have caused their disease (and thus remembering every detail about their use of oral contraceptives). In contrast, typically healthy women without breast cancer, who have no similar drive to ruminate about their history, may fail to remember the details of their exposure as accurately and thus may underreport their use of oral contraceptives. Cohort studies avoid this problem by securing exposure information prior to disease onset.

Women have worried for many years about the relationship of oral contraceptives to adverse health outcomes, and it seems difficult to believe that possible recent increases in levels of worry and awareness might affect recall and thus findings in recent studies. Also, although it is conceivable that this type of selective memory might operate with a fairly unmemorable exposure (e.g., aspirin use 10 years earlier), oral contraceptive use is so strongly linked with other reproductive experiences that it is unlikely that only in recent studies would controls have been underreporting their oral contraceptive use because of an inability to recall exposure.

3. Some other methodological problem(s) may have been introduced in these recent studies that have yet to be identified, although there is no evidence supporting this hypothesis.

4. These recent findings could simply be due to chance. The fact that there is some consistency to the positive findings, namely involving prolonged use at an early age, decreases our ability to attribute these findings to chance.

5. Little is known about the relationship between various formulations of the pill and breast cancer risk, largely because no reliable classification system of the effects on the breast of oral contraceptives and their components has been developed. Many of the women in the recent studies may well have been exposed to both high- and low-dose pills. Although removal of the high-dose pills successfully decreased deleterious cardiovascular and other side effects experienced by pill users, it is not actually known if the newer formulations are necessarily associated with a lower, higher, or unchanged risk of

breast cancer. It is possible that there are some aspects of oral contraceptive formulations whose effects on breast cancer risk have only recently become apparent.

6. Only studies of women born since the mid-1940s could have included large numbers of women exposed to oral contraceptives at a young age. Although no one is sure of the exact latency period for breast cancer, studies of atomic bomb survivors and the risk patterns observed in breast cancer for other factors such as menarche and age at first birth suggest a long latency period of at least 15 years. If hormones have a promotional effect, it is not yet known which time-related factors may be most relevant. Studies conducted in the latter half of the 1980s may be the first conducted in women born recently enough to have used oral contraceptives at a young age and for a long enough duration and whose use preceded the diagnosis of disease by a sufficient amount of time to be consistent with a latent period for breast carcinogenesis. Oral contraceptives may have a differential effect on young breast tissue, and this effect may just have become detectable in the more recent studies. Alternatively, the effect on young breast tissue may not translate into detectable breast cancer until 30 or more years later, in which case current studies will not be able to detect this association.

If risk increases in relation to use at an early age, recent findings supporting this premise may represent only the tip of the iceberg because the cohort of women who could have used the pill at an early age has yet to enter the highest breast cancer incidence age cohorts.

THE FUTURE

Many questions remain concerning the relationship between oral contraceptives and breast cancer risk. Gaining insight will entail a collaborative interdisciplinary effort by epidemiologists, clinicians, and basic scientists. Specific future endeavors could include some of the activities noted below.

Appropriate methods should be developed to classify the potency of oral contraceptives. More information is needed on the basic biology of estrogen and progestin as separate components as well as combined products. A better understanding is required of the biological effects of hormones on breast tissue. (Most past classification systems of hormonal effects have been based on effects on the endometrium.)

In the past decade, as the state of the art in epidemiological design has advanced, the criteria for what constitutes a methodologically suitable study have increased. A number of the studies reviewed here were plagued with limitations that, at the very least, render these studies suboptimal. Future case-control studies should be carefully designed so as to avoid some of these pitfalls. More work is needed to address the possibility of recall bias, although it is hard to believe that reporting of long-term use is compromised enough to explain the recent emergence of positive findings. Validation of a reported history of oral contraceptive use through medical record review would be ideal, but is quite difficult in the United States or any country where people are mobile and do not have a centralized source of health care. Case-control or small validation studies conducted in health maintenance organizations, or studies in countries with national health care systems, both of which have lifelong medical records for study subjects, might be the best way to evaluate the question of misclassification of oral contraceptive use because of recall bias. Future case-control studies should be population based, achieve high levels of response, and be designed to minimize the likelihood of introducing bias.

The causes of the increase in breast cancer incidence should be investigated further, and the extent to which increased breast screening contributes to the increased incidence should be evaluated. In turn, for case-control studies, the degree to which increased screening of oral contraceptive users affects case identification needs to be evaluated.

In existing and future data, especially those studies with large enough numbers of subjects, more effort is needed to tease out the effects of long duration of exposure versus exposure at specific ages—as well as other patterns of use that may be associated with adverse or protective effects. In particular, the effect of use at an early age should be further evaluated to distinguish the timing of exposure from the longer duration of exposure that is associated with beginning use at an earlier age. Besides examining oral contraceptive use at young ages, there are unanswered questions concerning use during the perimenopausal years. The recent FDA decision to lift the recommended upper age limit for use of oral contraceptives will probably lead to increased use in the over-40 age group. The relationship between oral contraceptives and breast cancer risk also needs to be examined in other subgroups, such as women with a strong family history of breast cancer and women with previous benign breast disease, using data sets with sufficient numbers of subjects.

In conclusion, the current picture of the relationship between oral contraceptives and breast cancer is rather confusing. It is not clear whether we should be reassured or alarmed, or whether it is just too early to know. Despite the more than 40 epidemiological studies conducted thus far, the end result seems to be more questions than answers.

REFERENCES

Brinton, L. A., R. Hoover, M. Szklo, and F. J. Fraumeni, Jr. 1982. Oral contraceptives and breast cancer. International Journal of Epidemiology 11:316-322.

(CASH) Cancer and Steroid Hormone Study of the Centers for Disease Control and the National Institute of Child Health and Human Development: Long-term oral contraceptive use and the risk of breast cancer. 1983. Journal of the American Medical Association 249:1591-1595.

Cancer and Steroid Hormone Study of the Centers for Disease Control and the National Institute of Child Health and Human Development: Oral-contraceptive use and the risk of breast cancer. 1986. New England Journal of Medicine 315(7):405-411.

Ellery, C., R. MacLennan, G. Berry, and R. P. Sherman. 1986. A case-control study of breast cancer in relation to the use of steroid contraceptive agents. Medical Journal of Australia 144:173-176.

Fasal, E., and R. S. Paffenbarger. 1975. Oral contraceptives as related to cancer and benign lesions of the breast. Journal of the National Cancer Institute 55:767-773.

Greenland, S. 1983. Tests for interaction in epidemiologic studies: A review and a study of power. Statistics in Medicine 2:243-251.

Harris, N. V., N. S. Weiss, A. M. Francis, and L. Polisar. 1982. Breast cancer in relation to patterns of oral contraceptive use. American Journal of Epidemiology 116:643-651.

Henderson, B. E., D. Powell, I. Rosario, et al. 1974. An epidemiologic study of breast cancer. Journal of the National Cancer Institute 53:609-614.

Hennekens, C. H., F. E. Speizer, R. J. Lipnick, B. Rosner, C. Bain, C. Belanger, M. Stampfer, W. Willett, and R. Peto. 1984. A case-control study of oral contraceptive use and breast cancer. Journal of the National Cancer Institute 72:39-42.

Janerich, D. T., A. P. Polednak, D. M. Glebatis, and C. E. Lawrence. 1983. Breast cancer and oral contraceptive use: A case-control study. Journal of Chronic Diseases 36(9): 639-646.

Jick, S. S., A. M. Walker, A. Stergachis, and H. Jick. 1989. Oral contraceptives and breast cancer. British Journal of Cancer 59:618-621.

Kay, C. R., and P. C. Hannaford. 1988. Breast cancer and the pill—A further report from the Royal College of General Practitioners' oral contraception study. British Journal of Cancer 58:675-680.

Kelsey, J. L., T. R. Holford, C. White, E. S. Mayer, S. E. Kilty, and R. M. Acheson. 1978. Oral contraceptives and breast disease. American Journal of Epidemiology 107:236-244.

Kelsey, J. L., D. B. Fischer, T. R. Holford, V. A. Livolsi, E. D. Moston, I. S. Goldenberg, and C. White. 1981. Exogenous estrogens and other factors in the epidemiology of breast cancer. Journal of the National Cancer Institute 67:327-333.

La Vecchia, C., A. Decarli, M. Fasoli, S. Franceschi, A. Gentile, E. Negri, F. Parazzini, and G. Tognoni. 1986. Oral contraceptives and cancers of the breast and the female reproductive tract. Interim results from a case-control study. British Journal of Cancer 54(2):311-317.

Lee, N. C., L. Rosero-Bixby, M. W. Oberle, C. Grimaldo, A. S. Whatley, and E. Z. Rovira. 1987. A case-control study of breast cancer and hormonal contraception in Costa Rica. Journal of the National Cancer Institute 79(6):1247-1254.

Lees, A. W., P. E. Burns, and M. Grace. 1978. Oral contraceptives and breast disease in premenopausal northern Albertan women. International Journal of Cancer 22:700-707.

Lipnick, R. J., J. E. Buring, C. H. Hennekens, B. Rosner, W. Willet, C. Bain, M. P. Stampfer, G. Colditz, R. Peto, and F. E. Speizer. 1986. Oral contraceptives and breast cancer: A prospective cohort study. Journal of the American Medical Association 255:58-61.

McPherson, K., and J. Drife. 1986. The pill and breast cancer: Why the uncertainty. British Medical Journal 293(6549):709.

McPherson, K., A. Neil, M. P. Vessey, and R. Doll. 1983. Oral contraceptives and breast cancer (letter). Lancet 12/17:1414-1415.

McPherson, K., M. P. Vessey, A. Neil, R. Doll, L. Jones, and M. Roberts. 1987. Early oral contraceptive use and breast cancer: Results of another case-control study. British Journal of Cancer 56:653-660.

Meirik, O., E. Lund, H. O. Adami, R. Bergstrom, T. Christofferson, and P. Bergsjo. 1986. Oral contraceptive use and breast cancer in young women. A joint national case-control study in Sweden and Norway. Lancet 2:650-654.

Meirik, O., T. M. Farley, E. Lund, H. O. Adami, T. Christoffersen, and P. Bergsjo. 1989. Breast cancer and oral contraceptives: Patterns of risk among parous and nulliparous women—further analysis of the Swedish-Norwegian material. Contraception39(5):471-475.

Miller, D. R., L. Rosenberg, D. W. Kaufman, D. Schottenfeld, P. D. Stolley, and S. Shapiro. 1986. Breast cancer risk in relation to early oral contraceptive use. Obstetrics and Gynecology 68:863-868.

Miller, D. R., L. Rosenberg, D. W. Kaufman, P. D. Stolley, M. E. Warshaver, and S. Shapiro. 1989. Breast cancer before age 45 and oral contraceptive use: New findings. American Journal of Epidemiology 129:269-280.

Murray, P. P., B. V. Stadel, and J. J. Schlesselman. 1989. Oral contraceptive use in women with a family history of breast cancer. Obstetrics and Gynecology 73:977-983.

Olsson, H., M. Landin-Olsson, T. Moller, J. Ranstam, and P. Holm. 1985. Oral contraceptive use and breast cancer in young women in Sweden. Lancet 30:748-749.

Olsson, H., T. R. Moller, and J. Ranstam. 1989. Early oral contraceptive use and breast cancer among premenopausal women: Final report from a study in southern Sweden. Journal of the National Cancer Institute 81(13):1000-1004.

Paffenbarger, R. S., J. B. Kambert, and H. G. Chang. 1980. Characteristics that predict risk of breast cancer before and after the menopause. American Journal of Epidemiology 112(2):258-268.

Paul, C., D. C. G. Skegg, G. H. Spears, and J. M. Kaldor. 1986. Oral contraceptives and breast cancer: A national study. British Medical Journal 293:723-726.

Peto, J. 1989. Oral contraceptives and breast cancer: Is the CASH study really negative? Lancet 1:552.

Pike, M. C., B. E. Henderson, J. T. Casagrande, I. Rosario, and G. E. Gray. 1981. Oral contraceptive use and early abortion as risk factors for breast cancer in young women. British Journal of Cancer 43:72-76.

Pike, M. C., B. E. Henderson, M. D. Krailo, and A. Duke. 1983. Breast cancer in young women and use of oral contraceptives: Possible modifying effect of formulation and age at use. Lancet 2:926-930.

Piper, J. M., and D. L. Kennedy. 1987. Oral contraceptives in the US: Trends in content and potency. International Journal of Epidemiology 16(2):215-221.

Ravnihar, B., D. G. Seigel, and J. Lindtner. 1979. An epidemiologic study of breast cancer and benign breast neoplasias in relation to the oral contraceptive and estrogen use. European Journal of Cancer 15:395-405.

Ravnihar, B., M. P. Zakelj, K. Kosmelj, and J. Stare. 1988. A case-control study of breast cancer in relation to oral contraceptive use in Slovenia. Neoplasma 35:109-121.

Romieu, I., W. C. Willett, G. A. Colditz, M. J. Stamfer, B. Rosner, C. H. Hennekens, and F. E. Speizer. 1989. Prospective study of oral contraceptive use and risk of breast cancer in women. Journal of the National Cancer Institute 81(17):1313-1321.

Rosenberg, L., D. R. Miller, D. W. Kaufman, S. P. Helmrich, P. D. Stolley, D. Schottenfeld, and S. Shapiro. 1984. Breast cancer and oral contraceptive use. American Journal of Epidemiology 119:167-176.

Royal College of General Practitioners. 1981. Breast cancer and oral contraceptives: Findings in Royal College of General Practitioners' Study. British Medical Journal 282:2089-2093.

Sartwell, P. E., F. G. Arthes, and J. A. Tonascia. 1977. Exogenous hormones, reproductive history and breast cancer. Journal of the National Cancer Institute 59:1589-1595.

Schlesselman, J. J., B. V. Stadel, P. Murray, S. Lai. 1987. Breast cancer in relation to type of estrogen contained in oral contraceptives. Contraception 36(6):595-612.

Schlesselman, J. J., B. V. Stadel, P. Murray, and S. Lai. 1988. Breast cancer in relation to early use of oral contraceptives: No evidence of a latency effect. Journal of the American Medical Association 259:1828-1833.

Smith, P. G., and N. E. Day. 1984. The design of case-control studies: The influence of confounding and interaction effects. International Journal of Epidemiology 13(3):356-365.

Spirtas, R. 1989. Breast cancer before age 45 and oral contraceptive use: New findings (letter). American Journal of Epidemiology 130:1255-1256.

Stadel, B. V., and J. J. Schlesselman. 1986. Oral contraceptive use and the risk of breast cancer in women with a prior history of benign breast disease. American Journal of Epidemiology 123(3):373-382.

Stadel, B. V., G. L. Rubin, L. A. Webster, J. J. Schlesselman, and P. A. Wingo. 1985. Oral contraceptives and breast cancer in young women. Lancet 2:970-973.

Stadel, B. V., S. Lai, J. J. Schlesselman, and P. Murray. 1988. Oral contraceptives and premenopausal breast cancer in nulliparous women. Contraception 38(3):287-299.

Stanford, J. L., L. A. Brinton, and R. N. Hoover. 1989. Oral contraceptives and breast cancer: Results from an expanded case-control study. British Journal of Cancer 60:375-381.

Talamini, R., C. La Vecchia, S. Franceschi, F. Colombo, et al. 1985. Reproductive, hormonal factors and breast cancer in a northern Italian population. International Journal of Epidemiology 14:70-74.

Thomas, D. B. 1984. Do hormones cause breast cancer? Cancer 53:595-604.

Trapido, E. J. 1981. A prospective study of oral contraceptives and breast cancer. Journal of the National Cancer Institute 67:1011-1015.

U.K. National Case-Control Study Group. 1989. Oral contraceptive use and breast cancer risk in young women. Lancet 8645:973-982.

Vessey, M. P., R. Doll, K. Jones, K. McPherson, and D. Yeates. 1979. An epidemiologic study of oral contraceptives and breast cancer. British Medical Journal 1:1755-1758.

Vessey, M. P., K. McPherson, and R. Doll. 1981. Breast cancer and oral contraceptives: Findings in the Oxford-Family Planning Association contraceptive study. British Medical Journal 282:2093-2094.

Vessey, M. P., K. McPherson, D. Yeates, and R. Doll. 1982. Oral contraceptive use and abortion before first term pregnancy in relation to cancer risk. British Journal of Cancer 45:327-331.

Vessey, M. P., J. Baron, R. Doll, K. McPherson, and D. Yeates. 1983. Oral contraceptives and breast cancer: Final report of an epidemiological study. British Journal of Cancer 47:455-462.

Vessey, M. P., K. McPherson, L. Villard-Mackintosh, and D. Yeates. 1989. Oral contraceptives and breast cancer: Latest findings in a large cohort study. British Journal of Cancer 59:613-617.

Yuan, J. M., M. C. Yu, R. K. Ross, Y. T. Gao, B. E. Henderson. 1988. Risk factors for breast cancer in Chinese women in Shanghai. Cancer Research 48:1949-1953.

(WHO) World Health Organization Collaborative Study of Neoplasia and Steroid Contraceptives. 1990. Breast cancer and combined oral contraceptives: Results from a multinational study. British Journal of Cancer 61:110-119.

B

Oral Contraceptives and Breast Cancer: Review of the Epidemiological Literature

DAVID B. THOMAS

Analysis of many of the risk factors for breast cancer suggests that endogenous ovarian hormones are of importance in the genesis of human mammary carcinomas. For example, risk is inversely related to age at menarche, and the younger a woman is at the time of her first full-term pregnancy, the lower her risk, suggesting that endocrinologic changes in a woman's early adult life can alter her susceptibility to breast cancer. Subsequent pregnancies after the first, and prolonged lactation, may reduce risk, whereas a first full-term pregnancy after about age 30 appears to enhance risk, suggesting that endocrinologic alterations during a woman's later reproductive years may also influence her risk. Finally, risk is inversely related to a woman's age at natural menopause or oophorectomy, indicating that endogenous hormonal changes late in reproductive life can have an impact on breast cancer development.

Because endogenous hormones presumably play an important role in breast cancer development, it is reasonable to ask whether exogenous hormones might also alter the risk of breast cancer. Unfortunately, the specific endocrinologic changes that mediate the various

David B. Thomas is professor of Epidemiology at the University of Washington and head of the Program in Epidemiology, Division of Public Health Sciences, at the Fred Hutchinson Cancer Research Center, Seattle, Washington.

risk factors for breast cancer are unknown; thus, it is impossible to predict a priori which exogenous hormonal preparations, if any, would be expected to enhance or reduce risk. It is reasonable, however, to suspect that the effects of these preparations on the risk of breast cancer may vary, depending on their compositions and the time during a woman's life when they are taken.

The purpose of this report is to critically review the results of epidemiologic studies of breast cancer in relation to combined oral contraceptives. Risk in relation to various features of use, and use at different times in a woman's life, are considered, as is use by women in various countries, and by women with and without other risk factors for breast cancer.

Sequential oral contraceptives contain only an estrogen for approximately two weeks of a cycle of daily use, and an estrogen-progestin combination for an additional week. These preparations have not been adequately studied in relation to breast cancer and are therefore not considered in this review. For the same reason, progestogen-only and triphasic pills are also not considered. Results of studies of benign breast lesions and oral contraceptives are also not included in this review. The author has, however, recently reviewed this topic (Thomas, 1989) and little new information has been published since that review was written.

METHODS

The author reviewed all reports known to him of case-control and cohort studies of breast cancer in relation to use of oral contraceptives and ascertained estimates of relative risks of breast cancer in relation to various measures of use from each study. When results of multiple studies of a particular exposure were available, the results of each were summarized in tabular form; when appropriate, if sufficient detail was available in the published reports, summary relative risks based on data from all relevant studies, and 95 percent confidence intervals of these summary relative risks, were estimated according to methods developed by Prentice (Prentice and Thomas, 1986). When these estimates were made, a chi-square test for heterogeneity of the estimates from the various studies was also performed. A statistically significant ($p < .05$) chi-square for heterogeneity suggests that the results of the summarized studies are not consistent and that nonbiological reasons for the variations in findings should be considered. Summary relative risks were calculated separately for case-control and cohort studies because these two investigative techniques are prone to different sources of bias.

RESULTS

Risk of Oral Contraceptive Users of All Ages
in Developed Countries

Table B-1 shows results from 15 case-control studies that were conducted in developed countries and included women of all ages who were at risk of prior exposure to oral contraceptives. Excluded from this table are studies that did not report results for women of all ages combined (Lubin et al., 1982; Mcpherson et al., 1987); studies that were part of a larger collaborative study (e.g., Ellery et al., 1986); a study that used women with benign breast disease as controls (Clavel et al., 1981); and reports of studies that have been updated by subsequent reports (e.g., Brinton et al., 1982). Only one of the studies summarized in Table B-1 found a relative risk of breast cancer in

TABLE B-1 Relative Risks of Breast Cancer in Women in Developed Countries Who Have Ever Used Oral Contraceptives: Case-Control Studies of Women of All Ages at Risk of Exposure

First Author (Date)	Upper Age Limit (years)	No. of Cases/Controls Users	Nonusers	Estimate of Relative Risk (Confidence Interval)[a]
Henderson (1974)	64	59/69	248/238	0.7[0.5,1.2]
Paffenbarger (1977)	50	226/398	226/474	1.1[0.9,1.4]
Sartwell (1977)	74	22/34	262/333	0.9(0.5,1.5)
Ravnihar (1979)	64	30/65	160/315	0.9[0.6,1.5]
Kelsey (1981)	74	30/141	300/1,207	0.9(0.6,1.3)
Harris (1982)	54	36/189	73/279	1.0(0.6,1.4)
Vessey (1983)	50	537/554	639/622	1.0(0.8,1.2)
Rosenberg (1984)	59	397/2,558	794/2,468	0.9(0.8,1.1)
Talamini (1985)	79	15/23	353/351	0.7(0.4,1.4)
CASH[b] (1986)	54	2,743/2,802	1,870/1,774	1.0(0.9,1.1)
Paul (1986)	54	310/708	123/189	0.9(0.7,1.3)
La Vecchia (1986)	60	104/178	672/1,104	1.1(0.8,1.5)
Ravnihar (1988)	54	162/467	372/1,522	1.6(1.3,2.1)
Stanford (1989)	>60	481/515	1,541/1,668	1.0(0.9,1.2)
WHO (1990)[c]	62	438/1,496	716/1,888	1.1(0.9,1.3)
Summary relative risk				1.0[1.0,1.1][d]

[a]Confidence interval of 95 percent used; [ ] = confidence intervals estimated from published data.
[b]CASH = Cancer and Steroid Hormone Study.
[c]WHO = World Health Organization.
[d]p value of chi-square test for heterogeneity = .08.

TABLE B-2 Relative Risks of Breast Cancer in Women Who Have Ever Used Oral Contraceptives: Cohort Studies

First Author (Date)	Upper Age Limit (years)	No. of Cases per 1,000 Person-Years		Estimate of Relative Risk (Confidence Interval)[a]
		"Ever" Users	"Never" Users	
Trapido (1981)[b]	>50	0.93 (85)	1.11 (370)	0.84(0.7,1.10)
Vessey (1981)[c]	45	0.50 (39)	0.52 (33)	0.96(0.59,1.63)
Kay (1988)[c]	64	0.64 (143)	0.52 (96)	1.22(0.93,1.60)
Romieu (1989)[d]	65	1.45 (717)	1.76 (1,041)	1.07(0.97,1.19)
Mills (1989)[e]	67	0.93 (29)	1.65 (64)	1.54(0.94,2.53)
Summary relative risk				
Excluding Mills (1989)				1.04[0.96,1.13][f]
Including Mills (1989)				1.06[0.97,1.15][g]

[a]Confidence interval of 95 percent used; [ ] confidence intervals estimated from published reports.
[b]Conducted in the Boston area.
[c]Study conducted in Britain.
[d]Nurses Health Study (U.S.A.)
[e]Conducted among Seventh Day Adventists (U.S.A.).
[f]p value of chi-square test for heterogeneity = .18.
[g]p value of chi-square test for heterogeneity = .13.

women who had ever used oral contraceptives that was significantly greater than 1.0 (Ravnihar et al., 1988), and the summary relative risk is close to unity, with narrow confidence limits. The variability of the relative risk estimates among studies was not statistically significant (p = .08).

Table B-2 summarizes relative risk estimates from five cohort studies of women who have ever used oral contraceptives. Results from the Vessey study (1981) have been updated (Vessey et al., 1989) but not reported for women of all ages combined, and the updated results therefore could not be included in this table, or in Tables B-4 and B-6. The study of Mills and colleagues (1989) was conducted among Seventh Day Adventists, who tend to have rates of breast cancer that are somewhat lower than women in the general U.S. population. Summary relative risks were therefore calculated with and without inclusion of data from that study. Both summary estimates are close to 1.0, with narrow confidence limits that barely include 1.0. The heterogeneity of the estimates from the individual studies could have occurred readily by chance. All of the relative risk estimates from the individual studies have 95 percent confidence intervals that include 1.0; although three are of borderline statistical significance.

TABLE B-3   Relative Risks of Breast Cancer in Long-term Users of Oral Contraceptives in Developed Countries: Case-Control Studies of Women of all Ages at Risk of Exposure

First Author (Date)	Mini- mum Years of Use	Age of Cases (years)	No. of Cases/Controls Long-term Users	Nonusers	Estimate of Relative Risk (Confidence Interval)[a]
Harris (1982)	5	35-54	17/99	73/279	0.8(0.5,1.4)
Ravnihar (1988)	7	25-54	34/66	372/1,522	2.4(1.5,3.8)[b]
Paffenbarger (1977)	8	<50	17/26	104/195	1.7[0.9,3.3]
Vessey (1983)	8	16-50	66/66	639/622	1.0(0.7,1.5)
WHO (1990)[c]	8	<62	89/206	716/1,888	1.4(1.0,1.9)
Rosenberg (1984)	10	20-59	25/128	794/2,468	0.8(0.5,1.3)
CASH[d] (1986)	15	20-54	45/69	1,870/1,774	0.6(0.4,0.9)
Paul (1986)	10	25-54	63/130	123/189	1.0[0.7,1.4]
Stanford (1989)	15	<40->60	8/13	1,541/1,668	0.7(0.3,1.6)
Summary relative risk					1.1[0.9,1.2][e]

[a]Confidence interval of 95 percent used; [ ] = confidence intervals estimated from published data.
[b]*p* value of test for trend of increasing risk with duration of use < .05. No significant trends were observed in other studies.
[c]WHO = World Health Organization; based on data from three developed countries only (Israel, German Democratic Republic, and Australia).
[d]CASH = Cancer and Steroid Hormone Study.
[e]*p* value of chi-square test for heterogeneity = .0005.

Table B-3 shows estimates from nine case-control studies of the relative risk of breast cancer in long-term users of oral contraceptiges. As in Table B-1, the studies shown are restricted to those in developed countries that include women of all ages at risk of exposure. The summary relative risk is not appreciably or significantly greater than 1.0, although there is considerable variation in results among the various studies. Only one study (Ravnihar et al., 1988) found a significant trend of increasing risk with duration of exposure.

Estimates of relative risks in long-term users from four cohort studies are shown in Table B-4. The results from the studies of Trapido (1981) and Romieu and colleagues (1989) refer to duration of use prior to entering the cohort, and do not include women who used oral contraceptives after the cohort was established. The Vessey study (1989) is not included in the table because results were not presented for women of all ages combined. As in Table B-2, summary relative risks are shown including and excluding results from the Seventh Day Adventist Study (Mills et al., 1989), although the numbers of long-term users in that study were too small to influence the value of the summary relative risk appreciably. A (nonsignificant) relative

TABLE B-4 Relative Risks of Breast Cancer in Long-term Users of Oral Contraceptives: Cohort Studies

First Author/Date	Mini- mum Years of Use	Upper Age Limit of Cases (years)	Cases per 1,000 Person-Years (No. of Cases)		Estimate of Relative Risk (Confidence Interval)[a]
			Long-term Users	Nonusers	
Trapido (1981)	5	>50	0.96 (15)	1.11 (370)	0.86[0.52,1.43]
Kay (1988)	10	65	0.75 (22)	0.52 (96)	1.44(0.91,2.29)
Romieu (1989)	10	65	1.73 (63)	1.76 (1,041)	1.09[0.84,1.41][b]
Mills (1989)	10	67	1.20 (2)	1.65 (64)	1.42(0.34,5.98)
Summary relative risk					
Excluding Trapido					1.17[0.94,1.46][c]
Excluding Mills					1.11[0.90,1.36][d]
No exclusions					1.11[0.91,1.36][e]

[a]Confidence interval of 95 percent used; [ ] = confidence intervals estimated from published data.
[b]Estimated by combining relative risks of 1.09(0.83,1.43) and 1.06(0.49,2.76) for users of 10-15 and >15 years, respectively.
[c]p value of chi-square test for heterogeneity = .57.
[d]p value of chi-square test for heterogeneity = .34.
[e]p value of chi-square test for heterogeneity = .52.

TABLE B-5 Relative Risks of Breast Cancer Long After Initial Use of Oral Contraceptives: Case-Control Studies of Women of All Ages for Risk of Exposure

First Author/ Date	Upper Age Limit of Cases (years)	Minimum Years Since First Use	No. of Cases/Controls		Estimate of Relative Risk (Confidence Interval)[a]
			Long-term Users	Nonusers	
Harris (1982)	54	15	15/45	73/279	1.4(0.8,2.4)
Vessey (1983)	50	12	112/154	639/622	0.7(0.5,1.0)
Rosenberg (1984)	59	15	101/347	794/2,468	1.1(0.9,1.4)
CASH[b] (1986)	54	20	Not given	1,872/1,774	0.8(0.7,1.0)
La Vecchia (1986)	60	10	63/72	672/1,104	1.5(1.0,2.1)
Paul (1986)	54	15	217/431	123/198	0.9[0.7,1.2]
Ravnihar (1988)	54	12	60/195	372/1,522	1.4(1.0,2.0)[c]
Stanford (1989)	>60	15	98/127	1,541/1,668	0.8(0.6,1.1)
WHO (1990)[d]	62	15	96/350	716/1,888	0.9(0.7,1.2)
Summary relative risk					1.0[0.9,1.1][e]

[a]Confidence interval of 95 percent used; [ ] = confidence intervals estimated from published data.
[b]CASH = Cancer and Steroid Hormone Study.
[c]p value of test for trend of increasing risk with duration of use = < .05. No significant trends observed in other studies.
[d]WHO = World Health Organization; based on data from three developed countries only (Israel, German Democratic Republic, and Australia).
[e]p value of chi-square test for heterogeneity = .004.

TABLE B-6   Relative Risks of Breast Cancer Long After Initial Use of Oral Contraceptives: Cohort Studies

First Author (Date)	Minimum Years Since First Use	Upper Age Limit of Cases (years)	Cases per 1,000 Persons (No. of Cases)		Estimate of Relative Risk (Confidence Interval)[a]
			Long-term Users	Nonusers	
Trapido (1981)	10	>50	1.13 (31)	1.11 (370)	1.0[0.7,1.5]
Vessey (1981)	12	45	0.82 (7)	0.52 (33)	1.6[0.7,3.6]
Kay (1988)	10	64	0.96 (17)	0.52 (96)	1.9(1.1,3.1)[b]
Romieu (1989)	20	65	1.75 (143)	1.76(1,041)	1.0(0.9,1.2)
Summary relative risk					1.1[0.9,1.3][c]

[a]Confidence interval of 95 percent used; [ ] = confidence intervals estimated from published data.
[b]p value of chi-square test for linear trend = .01. No significant trends were observed in other studies.
[c]p value of chi-square test for heterogeneity = .13.

risk of 1.11 in long-term users was estimated by combining results from all four studies. When results were considered only from the three studies that provided estimates in users of more than 10 years' duration, a combined relative risk of 1.17 was obtained; but the 95 percent confidence interval of this estimate also includes 1.0. The results of the four studies are not significantly heterogeneous. No significant trends of increasing risk with longer duration of use were observed in any of the studies.

Table B-5 summarizes results from nine case-control studies that attempted to assess risk long after initial exposure to combined oral contraceptives. No consistent increase in risk 10 to 20 years since first exposure is evident. The relative risks of 0.7 and 0.8 in the investigations by Vessey and colleagues (1983) and the Cancer and Steroid Hormone Study (1986), and of 1.4 in the studies by La Vecchia and coworkers (1986) and Ravnihar and colleagues (1988), were of borderline statistical significance; but only the Ravnihar study found a significant trend in risk with time since initial exposure. Although the summary relative risk is close to 1.0, the corresponding chi-square test for heterogeneity is statistically significant ($p < .05$), suggesting that caution should be exercised in interpreting this summary relative risk estimate. Results from three of four cohort studies (Table B-6) do not show a significant alteration in risk long after initial exposure to oral contraceptives, but one (Kay and Hannaford, 1988) found a significant trend of increasing risk with time since first use. The reasons for these discrepant findings are not known, but such varying results indicate that interpretations should be made with caution. In the aggregate, the information summarized in Tables B-5 and B-6 suggests that the use of oral contraceptives has not greatly influenced the risk of breast cancer in women of all ages combined, one to two decades after initial exposure.

Risk in Oral Contraceptive Users in Developing Countries

Results were recently published from a large hospital-based case-control study that was conducted primarily to determine whether possible relationships between oral contraceptives and breast (and other) cancers differ in developing and developed countries (World Health Organization [WHO], 1990). Such countries tend, respectively, to have relatively lower and higher rates of breast cancer. Based on data from three developed countries (Australia, German Democratic Republic, and Israel) and seven developing countries (Chile, Colombia, China, Kenya, Mexico, the Philippines, and Thailand), relative risks were found to be 1.07 (95 percent confidence interval (CI) = 0.91,1.26) and 1.24 (CI = 1.05,1.47), respectively, in women who had ever used oral contraceptives. The data also showed that women in developing countries had stronger trends of increasing risk with longer duration of use, and of decreasing risk with years since first or last exposure, than women in developed countries. Although it was concluded that a combination of chance and minor sources of bias and confounding could not be ruled out as the cause of the findings in developing countries, no specific reason for the results being spurious was identified, and a causal interpretation must also be considered.

Two smaller, population-based case-control studies in Costa Rica (Lee et al., 1987) and China (Yuan et al., 1988) yielded results that are not inconsistent with those of the WHO study. Results from all three investigations are summarized in Table B-7. Summary relative risks, based on data from the three studies, were estimated to be 1.21 (CI = 1.05,1.38) for "ever" users of oral contraceptives, and 1.59 (CI = 1.15,2.20) for long-term users (more than 8 to 10 years of use), respectively. The relative risk estimates from each of the three studies are not significantly heterogeneous. The relative risk for users of oral contraceptives that was observed in the Seventh Day Adventists Study (Mills et al., 1989), which was higher than those in other cohort studies (Table B-2), also supports the idea that relative risks of breast cancer in users of oral contraceptives are higher in low-risk than in high-risk populations.

TABLE B-7 Relative Risks of Breast Cancer in Users of Oral Contraceptives in Developing Countries: Summary of Three Case-Control Studies

First Author (Date)	Country	Cases/Controls			Relative Risk (Confidence Interval)[a]	
		Non-users	Ever Users	Long-term Users	Ever Use	Long-term Use
Lee (1987)	Costa Rica	97/427	58/321	6/29[b]	1.2 (0.8,1.8)	0.9 (0.4,2.6)
Yuan (1988)	China	435/439	99/95	16/12[b]	1.06 (0.74,1.51)	1.40 (0.62,3.17)
WHO[c] (1989)	Developing countries[d]	679/6,752	282/2,930	34/211[e]	1.24 (1.05,1.47)	1.88 (1.27,2.78)
Summary relative risk					1.21 [1.05,1.38][f]	1.59 [1.15,2.20][g]

[a]Confidence interval of 95 percent used; [ ] = confidence intervals estimated by approximate methods.
[b]Long-term = longer than 10 years.
[c]WHO = World Health Organization.
[d]Includes Chile, Colombia, China, Kenya, Mexico, the Philippines, and Thailand.
[e]Long-term = longer than 8 years.
[f]p value of chi-square test for heterogeneity = .43.
[g]p value of chi-square test for heterogeneity = .10.

Two possible biological reasons for these results have been proposed. One is that oral contraceptives could exert a small additive effect on risk, independent of the influence of other risk factors (WHO, 1990). Such an effect would give rise to higher relative risks in low-risk populations, even if the absolute increase in risk in users of oral contraceptives was the same in all populations. The other possible hypothesis, developed by Stalsberg and colleagues (1989), is that oral contraceptives enhance risk in low-risk populations by stimulating proliferation of the stem cells of the lobules; this phenomenon occurs to a greater extent in low risk populations (in which the lobular epithelium is not close to being maximally stimulated by other factors) than in high-risk populations (in which the lobular epithelium has reached its maximum proliferative capacity and thus cannot readily respond to the additional stimulus of exposure to oral contraceptives). In support of this hypothesis, Stalsberg and colleagues noted that tubular and lobular carcinomas, which probably arise from the lobular ductal epithelium, are more strongly related to oral contraceptives (and other presumably hormonally mediated risk factors) than are other histological types, which are more likely to arise from ductal epithelium.

Risk in Oral Contraceptive Users With and Without Various Risk Factors for Breast Cancer

If either of the above explanations for the possible higher relative risks of breast cancer among oral contraceptive users in low-risk populations is correct, then one might expect also to observe higher relative risks in women without other risk factors for breast cancer than in women with such risk factors. Alternatively, if oral contraceptives enhance risk by potentiating the effect of other risk factors, then one would expect to observe higher relative risks in users with the other risk factors than in users without them. Results from studies that assessed risk in users with and without various risk factors are in this section.

As shown in Table B-8, the WHO study (WHO, 1990) found a somewhat higher relative risk in users of low socioeconomic status (who tend to be at relatively low risk of breast cancer) than in women of higher status. This was not observed by Miller and colleagues (1989), however.

Nulliparous women tend to be at higher risk of breast cancer. Some nulliparous women are infertile and less likely than other women to use oral contraceptives; consequently, several studies (Table B-9), have assessed risk of breast cancer in relation to oral contraceptive use separately for nulliparous women. The results are inconsistent. Two studies found increasing risk with longer duration of use in young women (Stadel et al., 1989; U.K. National Case-Control Study Group, 1989), and another (Meirik et al., 1986) found significantly elevated relative risks in nulliparous women regardless of duration of use. Other equally well-designed and well-conducted studies, however, found no increase in risk in nulliparous users.

Risk of breast cancer increases with the age of a woman at the time of her first live birth. Table B-10 shows relative risks in relation to use of oral contraceptives in women of varying ages at the time of their first live birth. No trends of increasing or decreasing relative risk associated with age at first birth are seen in any study.

Women of high parity tend to be at low risk of breast cancer. Table B-11 shows that no studies have shown a trend in relative risks in users of oral contraceptives related to number of children that a woman has had.

Table B-12 shows relative risks in users of oral contraceptives who do and do not have a family history of breast cancer. None of the studies summarized showed appreciable differences in the magnitude of relative risks between women with and without various affected relatives.

Some studies have shown that obese women are at increased risk of breast cancer, especially in their postmenopausal years. As shown

TABLE B-8 Relative Risk of Breast Cancer in Women of Various Socioeconomic Strata Who Have Ever Used Oral Contraceptives

First Author (Date)	Measure of Socioeconomic Status	Level	Relative Risk	Confidence Interval (95%)
Miller (1989)	Years of education	<13	2.3	Includes 1.0[a]
		13-16	1.6	Includes 1.0
		≥17	2.8	Includes 1.0[b]
WHO[c] (1990)	Socioeconomic index[d]	4 (low)	1.86	1.07,3.24
		3	1.13	0.91,1.40
		2	1.14	0.94,1.39
		1 (high)	1.12	0.94,1.32

[a]In multivariate analysis, relative risk = 2.7 (95 percent confidence interval [CI] excludes 1.0).
[b]In multivariate analysis, relative risk = 3.9 (95 percent CI excludes 1.0).
[c]WHO = World Health Organization.
[d]Based on years of education and occupation.

TABLE B-9 Relative Risks of Breast Cancer in Nulliparous Women Who Have Ever Used Oral Contraceptives

First Author/Date (Study Design)	Restrictions on Study Population	Use of Oral Contraceptives	Estimate of Relative Risk (Confidence Interval)[a]
Paffenbarger/1977 (case-control)	15-39 years old	Any	4.6 /p = .16
	40-44 years old	Any	0.6 /p = .75
	45-49 years old	Any	0.8 /p = .99
	All ages	Any	1.1 /p = .99
Trapido/1981 (cohort)	None	Any	2.1(0.9,5.0)
Harris/1982 (case-control)	None	Any	0.8(0.2,2.6)
Hennekens/1984 (cohort)	None	Any	1.0(0.6,1.8)
Rosenberg/1984 (case-control)	None	<1 year	1.2(0.6,2.3)
		1-4 years	0.8(0.4,1.6)
		≥5 years	1.1(0.6,2.3)
		Any	1.1(0.7,1.7)
La Vecchia/1986 (case-control)	None	Any	1.16 (N.G.)[d]
Miller/1986 (case-control)	<45 years old	Any	1.0(0.2,3.9)
Kay/1988 (cohort)	None	Any	1.14(0.72,1.8)
Meirik/1989 (case-control)	<45 years old	<4 years	2.8(1.1,7.4)
		4-7 years	1.0(0.3,3.3)
		≥8 years	4.3(1.4,13.1)
Stadel/1989 (case-control)	20-44 years old	≤3 years	1.2(0.8,1.8)
		4-7 years	1.7(1.0,2.8)
		8-11 years	1.6(0.9,2.8)
		≥12 years	2.5(0.9,6.7)
	45-54 years old	≤3 years	0.6(0.3,1.1)
		4-7 years	1.2(0.2,6.0)
		8-11 years	0.3(0.0,1.6)
		≥12 years	0.3(0.1,1.4)
Stanford/1989 (case-control)	None	Any	0.89(0.5,1.4)
U.K. National Case-Control Study Group/ 1989 (case-control)	<36 years old	1-3 years	0.981 (N.G.)[b]
		4-8 years	1.37 (N.G.)
		≥9 years	2.30 (N.G.)
WHO[c] /1990 (case-control)	None	Any	0.84(0.56,1.25)

[a]Confidence interval of 95 percent used.
[b]p value of test for trend = .005.
[c]WHO = World Health Organization.
[d]NG = Not given.

TABLE B-10　Relative Risks of Breast Cancer in Parous Women Who Have Ever Used Oral Contraceptives by Age at First Live Birth

First Author/Date	Age in Years at First Live Birth			
(Study Design)	<20	20-24/<24	25-29/>25	>30
Trapido/1981	0.5	0.7	1.2	0.6
(cohort)				
Miller/1989	2.9[a]	2.1[a]	2.6[a]	N.a.
(case-control)				
Stanford/1989	0.74	0.93	1.09	1.04
(case-control)				
WHO[b]/1990	N.a.	1.17	1.27	1.13
(case-control)				

N.a: Not available.
[a]Confidence intervals of 95 percent exclude 1.0.
[b]WHO = World Health Organization.

in Table B-13, Miller and colleagues (1989) observed a trend of increasing relative risks in relation to oral contraceptive use with increasing body mass index. This trend was not observed by Stanford and colleagues (1989). The former study was restricted to women under age 45, when obesity has a minimal impact on risk of breast cancer; the latter study included older women.

Table B-14 shows the results of studies that assessed risk of breast cancer in oral contraceptive users with a history of benign breast disease. Risks were elevated in all three studies that confined analyses to young women (Lees et al., 1978; Paffenbarger et al., 1980; Janerich et al., 1983) with two of the studies showing an increasing risk with

TABLE B-11　Relative Risks of Breast Cancer in Women Who Have Ever Used Oral Contraceptives by Number of Children

First Author/Date	Number of Children				
(Study Design)	0	1/≥1	1-2	2-3/≥3	>4
La Vecchia/1986	1.16	1.00	N.a.	N.a.	N.a.
(case-control)					
Kay/1988	1.14	5.88[a]	N.a.	1.01	0.71
(cohort)					
Miller/1989	N.a.	N.a.	2.4[a]	2.9[a]	N.a.
(case-control)					

N.a.: Not available.
[a]Confidence intervals of 95 percent exclude 1.0.

TABLE B-12 Relative Risks of Breast Cancer in Relation to Use of Oral Contraceptives in Women With and Without a Family History of Breast Cancer

First Author/Date (Study Design)	Restrictions on Study Population	Relative with Breast Cancer	Use of Oral Contraceptives	Estimate of Relative Risk (Confidence Interval)[a]
Kelsey/1981 (case-control)	None	Any	Any	No increase (data not given)
Vessey/1983 (case-control)	None	Any	None	1.0
			≤48 mo	0.6
			>49 mo	1.1
Hennekens/1984 (case-control)	None	Not mother	Any	1.1(0.9,1.2)
		Mother	Any	1.0(0.6,1.7)
		Not sister	Any	1.1(0.9,1.3)
		Sister	Any	1.4(0.7,3.0)
Rosenberg/1984 (case-control)	None	Any	>5 yr	0.9(0.4,2.1)
CASH[b]/1986 (case-control)	None	None	Any	1.0(0.9,1.2)
		First degree	Any	1.1(0.8,1.6)
		Second degree	Any	0.9(0.7,1.2)
Lipnick/1986 (cohort)	None	Mother	Any	0.8(0.4,1.6)
		Sister	Any	0.9(0.5,1.5)
Miller/1989 (case-control)	<45 yr old	None	Any	2.0(includes 1.0)
		Any	Any	1.9(includes 1.0)[c]
Stanford/1989 (case-control)	None	Not mother	Any	1.0(0.8,1.2)
		Mother	Any	0.8(0.5,1.2)
		Not sister	Any	1.1(0.9,1.4)
		Sister	Any	1.2(0.6,2.5)
WHO[b]/1990 (case-control)	None	None	Any	1.1(1.01,1.27)
		Any	Any	1.3(0.75,2.16)

[a]Confidence interval of 95 percent used.
[b]CASH = Cancer and Steroid Hormone Study; WHO = World Health Organization.
[c]Relative risk = 3.4 in multivariate analysis (95 percent confidence interval includes 1.0).

duration of use. Pike and colleagues (1981) confined their analyses of data from young women to use of oral contraceptives before a woman's first pregnancy. They found risk associated with such use to be particularly high in women with a history of benign breast disease. On the other hand, no trends of risk increasing with duration of use were observed by Paffenbarger and colleagues (1980) in postmenopausal women, or by Vessey and coworkers (1983) or Rosenberg and colleagues (1984) in studies that were not confined to young women. Because young women tend to have fibroadenomas, whereas older

TABLE B-13 Relative Risk of Breast Cancer in Women with Varying Body Mass Indices Who Have Ever Used Oral Contraceptives

First Author (Date)	Body Mass Index[a]	Relative Risk	Confidence Interval (95%)
Miller (1989)	<21	1.6	Includes 1.0
	21-25	1.8	Includes 1.0
	≥26	3.5[b]	Includes 1.0
Stanford (1989)	<21	0.80	0.5,1.3
	22-23	0.89	0.6,1.2
	24-25	0.94	0.7,1.3
	≥26	0.88	0.5,1.5

[a]Weight (in kilograms)/height (in centimeters)^2.
[b]Relative risk = 4.2 (95 percent confidence interval excludes 1.0) in multivariate analysis.

women tend to have various forms of fibrocystic disease, these findings suggest that oral contraceptives may enhance the risk of breast cancer in women with specific histological types of benign lesions. No studies have been completed that assess risk of breast cancer in users with benign lesions and include as part of the investigation an independent review of slides from the benign lesions. Such studies are in progress, however.

Because oral contraceptives apparently protect against benign breast lesions, the assessment of the risk of breast cancer in users of oral contraceptives with prior benign lesions becomes complex. Stadel and Schlesselman (1986) have reviewed this issue and sensibly suggest that only oral contraceptive use after diagnosis of benign lesions should be considered when determining whether risk of breast cancer in women with benign breast disease is enhanced by use of oral contraceptives. This has been done in three studies summarized in Table B-15. None found an increased risk of breast cancer in women who took oral contraceptives after developing a benign breast lesion. None of these three studies are confined to young women.

Risk in Relation to Early Use of Oral Contraceptives

Because early menarche is associated with increased risk, and risk is reduced by an early first full-term pregnancy, it is reasonable to ask whether oral contraceptives used early in a woman's life, or before her first pregnancy, alter her risk of breast cancer. In 1981, Pike and colleagues confirmed earlier findings of Paffenbarger and col-

TABLE B-14 Relative Risks of Breast Cancer in Relation to Use of Oral Contraceptives in Women with Benign Breast Diseases: Case-Control Studies

First Author (Date)	Restrictions on Study Population	Use of Oral Contraceptives	Estimate of Relative Risk
Lees (1978)	30-49 yrs of age	None	1.0
		≤12 mo	1.0 (p>.05)
		13-59 mo	2.3 (p>.05)
		≥60 mo	9.2 (p<.02)
Paffenbarger (1980)	Premenopausal	None	1.0
		1-24 mo	0.5 (p>.05)
		25-48 mo	3.0 (p>.05)
		49-72 mo	1.2 (p>.05)
		≥73 mo	3.2 (p>.05)
	Postmenopausal	None	1.0
		1-24 mo	2.9 (p>.05)
		25-48 mo	1.0 (p>.05)
		49-72 mo	1.0 (p>.05)
		≥73 mo	0.8 (p>.05)
Kelsey (1978, 1981)	None	Any	No increase (data not given)
Janerich (1983)	<45 yrs	Any	2.5(1.1,5.3)[a]
Vessey (1983)	None	None	1.0
		≤48 mo	0.7
		≥49 mo	0.7
Rosenberg (1984)	None	>5 yrs	0.8(0.4,1.7)[a]

[a]( ) = Confidence interval of 95 percent.

leagues (1980) that in women young enough to have used the pill before their first full-term pregnancy, risk increased with duration of use before that event. (Table B-16 summarizes results from these and subsequent investigations of this issue.) Four additional studies (Harris et al., 1982; McPherson et al., 1986; U.K. National Case-Control Study Group, 1989; Lund et al., 1989) showed strong trends of increasing risk with duration of use before a woman's first full-term pregnancy, and six others (Stadel et al., 1985; Miller et al., 1986; Jick et al., 1989; Miller et al., 1989; Olsson et al., 1989; WHO, 1990) showed weaker associations between such use and breast cancer that were not statistically significant. Conversely, four studies (Vessey et al., 1982; Rosenberg et al., 1984; Paul et al., 1986; Stanford et al., 1989) found no association between use before a first birth and breast cancer. The results from Stanford and colleagues (1989) are not presented in Table B-16 because they were not published in tabular form.

A summary relative risk estimate of 1.44 (CI = 1.23,1.69) in long-term users before their first birth was obtained by combining results from all studies shown in the table. There is significant heterogeneity of results among studies, however, and this summary estimate should therefore be interpreted with caution. Table B-17 shows results from two cohort studies that are generally not supportive of this association. The reasons for the discrepant results are not known. Both population-based and hospital-based case-control studies of equally rigorous design have yielded conflicting results. Only the study by Olsson and coworkers (1989) has an obvious potential bias; in that study, physicians interviewed cases in the hospital, and interviewers interviewed controls in their homes by telephone.

McPherson and colleagues (1986) have suggested that the reason for the discrepant findings is that the studies that showed no association were unable to assess risk after a long potential latent period. As shown in Table B-18, however, four studies have shown that risk is not particularly enhanced more than a decade after exposure to oral contraceptives before a first birth (McPherson et al., 1987; Vessey et al., 1989; Paul et al., 1990) or after 15 years following the first birth in women who used the pill prior to that birth (Schlesselman et al., 1988).

It should also be noted that in two of the studies in Table B-16

TABLE B-15   Relative Risk of Breast Cancer in Women Who Used Oral Contraceptives Before and After Diagnosis of a Benign Breast Lesion

		Estimate of Relative Risk (Confidence Interval)[a]	
First Author (Date)	Use of Oral Contraceptives	Before Benign Breast Disease	After Benign Breast Disease
CASH[b] (1986)	Any	0.7(0.5,0.97)	0.8(0.5,1.2)
Stanford (1989)	Any	1.22(0.7,2.1)	0.87(0.6,1.3)
	≤5 years	1.48(0.8,2.7)	0.91(0.5,1.5)
	>5 years	0.55(0.2,1.7)	0.80(0.4,1.5)
WHO[b] (1990)	Any	1.30(0.75,2.27)	0.97(0.54,1.72)
Summary relative risk	Any	0.90[0.70,1.16][c]	0.86[0.66,1.12][d]

[a]Confidence interval of 95 percent used; [ ] = confidence intervals estimated by approximate methods.
[b]CASH = Cancer and Steroid Hormone Study; WHO = World Health Organization.
[c]*p* value of chi-square test for heterogeneity = .08.
[d]*p* value of chi-square test for heterogeneity = .87.

TABLE B-16 Relative Risks of Breast Cancer in Relation to Duration of Use of Oral Contraceptives Before First Full-term Pregnancy: Case-Control Studies

First Author (Date)	Ages of Cases at Diagnosis	Months of Use	No. of Subjects Cases	No. of Subjects Controls	Estimate of Relative Risk (Confidence Interval)[a]	p Value of Test for Trend
Paffenbarger (1980)	Premenopausal	0	57	1,146	1.0	Not given
		11-17	12	9	2.6[1.1,5.9]	
		≥18	18	16	2.6[1.3,4.0]	
Pike (1981)	<32	0	79	141	1.0	
		1-48	53	103	1.0[0.6,1.5]	.009
		≥49	31	26	2.5(1.4,4.5)	
Harris (1982)	35-54	<12	61	249	1.0	
		13-48	4	12	3.8(1.3,11.3)	.01
		≥49	1	1	12.9(0.6,265.6)	
Vessey (1982)	16-50	0	995	996	1.0	
		1-12	28	25	0.8[0.5,1.4]	
		13-48	18	22	0.7[0.4,1.5]	
		≥49	8	6	0.9[0.3,2.3]	
Rosenberg (1984)	<59	0	643	1,946	1.0	
		≤12	14	149	0.8(0.4,1.5)	>.05
		13-35	21	133	1.3(0.7,2.3)	
		≥36	10	91	0.9(0.4,1.8)	
Stadel (1985)	<44	0	Not given	Not given	1.0	
		≤12			1.3(1.0,1.7)	>.05
		13-48			1.1(0.9,1.5)	
		≥49			1.2(0.9,1.6)	
Miller (1986)	<45	0	209	214	1.0	>.05
		<12	35	41	0.7(0.4,1.2)	
		13-24	46	33	1.4(0.7,2.6)	
		25-48	26	25	0.8(0.4,1.6)	
		49-72	22	12	1.5(0.6,4.0)	
		≥73	18	15	1.4(0.6,3.2)	
Paul (1986)	25-54	0	268	472	1.0	.14
		<24	60	147	0.9[0.6,1.2]	
		24-47	26	82	0.8[0.5,1.3]	
		48-71	11	41	0.7[0.4,1.4]	
		≥72	11	52	0.6[0.3,1.1]	
McPherson et al. (1987)	<45	0	235	273	1.0	<.01
		1-12	27	26	1.0(0.5,1.9)	
		13-48	43	29	2.0(1.0,3.8)	
		≥48	46	23	2.6(1.3,5.4)	
Jick (1989)	<43	0	48	75	1.0	.2
		<12	1	4	0.3(0.0,3.5)	
		12-47	15	29	0.8(0.3,2.0)	
		≥48	12	11	1.3(0.3,4.6)	
Lund (1989) Sweden	<44	0	51	56	1.0	Not given
		≤47	73	71	1.1(0.7,1.9)	
		48-95	32	33	1.0(0.6,2.0)	
		≥96	13	10	1.5(0.6,3.9)	

TABLE B-16   (Continued)

First Author (Date)	Ages of Cases at Diagnosis	Months of Use	No. of Subjects Cases	No. of Subjects Controls	Estimate of Relative Risk (Confidence Interval)[a]	p Value of Test for Trend
Norway	<40	0	30	67	1.0	Not given
		≤47	19	30	1.4(0.6,3.0)	
		≥48	6	5	1.8[0.6,5.1][b]	
Miller (1989)	<45	0	85	109	1.0	Not given
		<12	27	21	1.5(0.7,3.7)	
		12-59	59	32	2.5(1.2,5.2)	
		≥69	14	12	1.3(0.4,4.0)	
Olsson	Premeno-	0	91	305	1.0	<.08
(1989)	pausal	<36	38	71	1.8(1.0,3.2)	
		37-95	30	58	2.1(1.1,3.8)	
		≥96	13	21	2.0(0.8,4.7)	
U.K. National Case-Control Study Group (1989)	<36	0	247	259	1.0	.02
		1-48	219	254	1.0[0.8,1.3]	
		49-96	112	88	1.5[1.4,2.1]	
		≥97	17	15	1.4[0.7,2.9]	
WHO[c] (1990)	<62	0	1,691	9,660	1.00	Not given
		<24	56	405	0.8(0.6,1.1)	
		≥24	29	110	1.2(0.8,2.0)	
Summary relative risk		Longest			1.4[1.2,1.7][d]	

[a]Confidence interval of 95 percent used; [ ] = confidence intervals estimated from published data.
[b]Calculated by combining relative risks of 2.2(0.5,9.8) and 1.4(0.1,26.7) for users of 48-95 and >96 months of use before their first full-term pregnancy.
[c]WHO = World Health Organization.
[d]p value of chi-square test for heterogeneity = .05.

(Miller et al., 1989; U.K. National Case-Control Study Group, 1989), equally strong associations were observed between risk of breast cancer and use after a woman's first live birth. In addition, in 1983 Pike and coworkers published an update of their earlier study. They did not present data on use before a first full-term pregnancy, but claimed that use at an early age (regardless of whether before or after first pregnancy) was more important than use before a first full-term pregnancy in increasing the risk of breast cancer. They reported an increase in risk with duration of use before the age of 25.

As shown in Table B-19, findings similar to those of Pike and colleagues (1983) were observed by Olsson and colleagues (1989), and to a lesser extent also by Meirik and coworkers (1986) and the WHO

TABLE B-17 Relative Risks of Breast Cancer in Relation to Duration of Use of Oral Contraceptives Before First Full-term Pregnancy: Cohort Studies

First Author (Date)	Months of Use	Cases per 1,000 Person-Years (No. of Cases)	Estimate of Relative Risk (Confidence Interval)[a]
Vessey (1989)[b]	0	0.57 (84)	1.00
	≤47	0.83 (15)	1.46[0.84,2.53]
	≥48	0.62 (7)	1.09[0.51,2.34]
Romieu (1989)[c]	0	1.60 (371)	1.00
	1-11	1.00 (52)	0.98(0.72,1.35)
	12-35	1.01 (34)	1.12(0.77,1.63)
	≥36	0.81 (9)	0.84(0.43,1.66)
Summary relative risk	Longest		0.94[0.57,1.55][d]

[a]Confidence interval of 95 percent used; [ ] = confidence intervals estimated from published data.
[b]Rates are age adjusted.
[c]Rates are not age adjusted.
[d]p value of chi-square test for heterogeneity = .62.

study (1990). The CASH (1986) study yielded equivocal results, with increased relative risks in some categories of years of use, but no trend of increasing risk with duration of exposure before age 25. Conversely, two studies (Miller et al., 1986; Paul et al., 1986) found no association between breast cancer and use before age 25.

Other investigators of early use did not publish their findings in such a manner that they could be included in Table B-19. McPherson and colleagues (1987) did not find an association with duration of use before age 25, but they did not publish relative risk estimates. Stanford and coworkers (1989) estimated the relative risk to be 0.96 (0.6,1.7) in women who had ever used oral contraceptives before age 25; this estimate, however, was based on only 26 exposed cases and 30 exposed controls, all of whom used oral contraceptives for less than five years before the age of 25. One cohort study (Vessey et al., 1989) found relative risks of 0.92 and 1.21 in women who had used oral contraceptives before age 25 for less than four years and for four or more years, respectively (based on 17 and 1 exposed cases, respectively). Thus, results from studies not included in Table B-19, like those shown in the table, have also yielded inconsistent results.

Other investigators have not presented results specifically for users before the age of 25, but have nevertheless published results that are broadly compatible with early oral contraceptive use being a risk factor for breast cancer. Miller and coworkers (1989) found increased risks in women who used the pill for more than five years in each of four age categories under the age of 44, and the U.K. National Case-Control Study Group (1989) found increasing risks with duration of use in women under age 36 who first used the pill at various ages. Because the authors of these studies (and some others summarized in Tables B-16, B-20, and B-21, but not included in Table B-19) did not specifically publish results of use before age 25, the reports that have

TABLE B-18 Relative Risks of Breast Cancer in Relation to Duration of Use of Oral Contraceptives Before a Woman's First Full-term Pregnancy, After Varying Potential Latent Periods

First Author (Date)[a]	Months of Use Before First Full-term Pregnancy	Excluding Use Before First Full-term Pregnancy Within the Following Years Prior to Diagnosis				
		No Exclusions	6 Years	10 Years	14 Years	20 Years
McPherson (1987)	0	1.00	1.00	1.00	1.00	
	1-12	1.02	1.24	1.20	1.74	
	13-48	1.97	1.83	2.45	1.37	
	>48	2.59	2.30	1.65	1.97	
Vessey (1989)	0	1.00	1.00	1.00		
	1-12	0.48	0.46	0.72		
	13-47	1.66	1.40	2.44		
	≥48	1.18	1.03	0.87		
Paul (1990)[b]	0	1.00	1.00	1.00	1.00	1.00
	<24	0.89	0.89	0.83	0.80	0.49
	25-47	0.81	0.81	0.86	0.96	2.0
	≥48	0.60	0.65	0.44	0.43	
Schlesselman (1988)[c]	0	1.0	1.0	1.0	1.0	
	<2	0.6	0.9	1.3	1.0	
	2-3	0.5	1.2	1.4	1.0	
	4-6	0.7	0.9	1.0	1.0	
	>6	0.6	0.7	1.1		

[a]All studies are case-control designs except Vessey, which is a cohort design.
[b]In this research periods of 5 years (rather than 6) and 15 years (rather than 14) were used.
[c]The Schlesselman study reported on years from first full-term pregnancy to diagnosis. Categories used were 0-4 years (rather than "No Exclusions"), 5-9 years (rather than "6 Years"), 10-14 years (rather than "10 Years"), and longer than 15 years (rather than "14 Years").

TABLE B-19 Relative Risks of Breast Cancer in Relation to Duration of Use of Oral Contraceptives Before Age 25: Case-Control Studies

First Author (Date)	Ages of Cases at Diagnosis	Months of Use	No. of Subjects Cases	Controls	Estimate of Relative Risk (Confidence Interval)[a]	p Value of Test for Trend
Pike (1983)	<37	0	65	93	1.0	<.0001
		<2	106	118	1.3(0.8,2.0)	
		2-3	79	67	1.7(1.0,2.7)	
		4-5	40	29	2.0(1.1,3.6)	
		≥6	24	7	4.9(1.9,13.4)	
Meirik (1986)	≤44	0	177	242	1.0	Not given
		<3	186	228	1.1(0.8,1.5)	
		4-7	51	54	1.1(0.7,1.8)	
		≥8	8	3	2.7(0.7,11.0)	
Paul (1986)	25-54	0	292	465	1.0	.4
		<2	81	191	1.2[1.0,1.5]	
		2-3	44	141	1.0[0.7,1.4]	
		4-5	11	65	0.7[0.4,1.3]	
		≥6	5	35	0.6[0.3,1.4]	
CASH (1986)[b]	≤44	0	257	259	1.0	Not sig.
		1-2	395	395	1.3(1.0,1.6)	
		3-4	266	267	1.3(1.0,1.8)	
		5-6	113	110	1.5(1.1,2.1)	
		>6	17	30	1.0(0.5,2.0)	
Miller (1986)	<45	0	207	214	1.0	Not sig.
		<1	26	35	0.8(0.4,1.5)	
		1-2	59	56	1.0(0.6,1.6)	
		3-4	43	33	1.3(0.7,2.3)	
		≥5	14	16	1.1(0.4,2.9)	
Olsson (1989)	Premeno-pausal	0	87	286	1.0	<.001
		<2	35	85	1.6(0.9,2.8)	
		3-5	34	69	2.0(1.1,3.5)	
		>5	15	19	5.3(2.1,13.2)	
WHO[c] (1990)	<62	0	1,908	11,104	1.0	.31
		<1	82	881	1.0(0.7,1.3)	
		1-2	37	421	0.8(0.6,1.1)	
		2-3	29	207	1.5(1.0,2.3)	
		>3	29	243	1.5(1.0,2.3)	
Summary relative risk		Longest			1.5[1.2,2.0][d]	

[a]Confidence interval of 95 percent used; [ ] = confidence intervals estimated from published data.
[b]CASH = Cancer and Steroid Hormone Study. Unpublished data provided by P. Wingo.
[c]WHO = World Health Organization.
[d]p value of chi-square test for heterogeneity = .002.

TABLE B-20   Relative Risks of Breast Cancer in Women Under 45 Years of Age Who Have Ever Used Oral Contraceptives: Summary of Results from Case-Control Studies

First Author (Date)	Age of Cases	Cases/Controls Nonusers	Users	Estimate of Relative Risk (Confdence Interval)[a]
Kelsey (1978)	20-44	59/65	40/34	1.6(0.8,2.4)
Vessey (1983)	≤45	N.g.[b]	N.g.[b]	0.81[0.6,1.03][c]
Janerich (1983)	≤45	120/264	133/233	1.22(0.88,1.69)
Rosenberg (1984)	20-39	68/872	149/1,804	1.13[0.78,1.63][c]
Paul (1986)	25-44	26/69	165/501	0.97[0.63,1.50][c]
Miller (1986)	<45	207/214	314/307	0.9(0.7,1.4)
Lee (1987)	25-44	27/225	37/273	1.15[0.7,2.0][c]
Ravnihar (1988)	25-44	112/556	115/345	1.64[1.19,2.26][c]
Jick (1989)	<43	28/29	78/124	0.9(0.4,1.9)
Miller (1989)	<45	125/176	282/248	2.0(1.4,2.9)
Stanford (1989)	<45	112/144	172/183	1.13[0.7,1.85][c]
WHO[d] (1990)	<35	141/2,722	160/1,613	1.26(0.95,1.66)
CASH[e]	<45	387/403	1,654/1,619	1.14(0.96,1.35)
Summary relative risk				1.16[1.05,1.28][f]

[a]Confidence interval of 95 percent used; [ ] = confidence interval estimated from published data.
[b]N.g. = number not given.
[c]Relative risk estimated by combining results from more than one age group under 45 years.
[d]WHO = World Health Organization.
[e]CASH = Cancer and Steroid Hormone Study. Unpublished data provided by P. Wingo.
[f]p value of chi-square test for heterogeneity = .006.

included such results may be biased in favor of including a disproportionate number with positive findings. Because of this likelihood and the significant heterogeneity of results among the studies in Table B-19 (and among those not included in this table), the summary relative risk of 1.53 (CI = 1.16,2.02) for long-term users before the age of 25 should be interpreted with caution.

Studies of breast cancer in relation to use of oral contraceptives at an early age have, of necessity, been confined largely to breast cancer in young women because the pill was not available when older women with breast cancer were in their early reproductive years. However, focusing attention on early use, rather than the effect of any long-term use on risk of breast cancer in young women, may have obscured underlying consistencies of results among studies. Table B-20 shows estimates from 13 studies of the relative risk of breast cancer in women under age 45 who have ever used oral contraceptives.

TABLE B-21 Relative Risks of Breast Cancer in Women Under 45 Years of Age with Long-term Oral Contraceptive Use: Summary of Results from Case-Control Studies

First Author (Date)	Age of Cases	Years of Use	Cases/Controls Nonusers	Users	Estimate of Relative Risk (Confidence Interval)[a]
Kelsey (1978)	20-44	>5	59/65	9/6	1.7 (0.5,5.4)
Janerich (1983)	<45	≥6	120/264	36/64	1.18 (0.94,1.45)
Rosenberg (1984)	20-39	>5	68/872	42/398	1.25 [0.84,1.85][b]
Meirik (1986)	<45	>12	96/156	39/23	2.2 (1.2,4.0)
Miller (1986)	<45	≥7	207/214	18/15	1.4 (0.6,3.2)
Paul (1986)	25-44	≥10	26/69	32/83	1.10 [0.60,2.04][c]
McPherson (1987)	<45	>12	111/122	21/20	1.78 (0.82,3.87)
Jick (1989)	<43	≥10	28/29	17/15	1.4 (0.4,4.6)
Miller (1989)	<45	≥10	125/176	26/16	4.1 (1.8,9.3)
U.K. National Case-Control Study Group (1989)	<36	>8	67/80	198/143	1.74 [1.29,2.33]
WHO[d] (1990)	<35	≥4	5/292	141/27,224	1.45 (0.97,2.21)[e]
CASH[f]	<45	≥10	387/403	205/174	1.23 (0.97,1.56)[g]
Summary relative risk					1.42 [1.25,1.63][h]

[a]Confidence interval of 95 percent used; [ ] = confidence interval estimated from published data.
[b]Value computed by combining relative risks of 0.8 and 1.3 in women in the age groups 20-29 and 30-39 years.
[c]Value computed by combining relative risks of 4.6 and 0.84 in women in the age groups 25-34 and 35-44 years.
[d]WHO = World Health Organization.
[e]Value computed by combining relative risks of 1.60 and 0.93 for users of 4-8 and >8 years, respectively.
[f]CASH = Cancer and Steroid Hormone Study. Unpublished data provided by P. Wingo.
[g]Value computed by combining relative risks of 1.28 and 0.93 for users of 10-14 years and >15 years, respectively.
[h]p value of chi-square test for heterogeneity = .21.

Although the 95 percent confidence interval of the summary relative risk does not include 1.0, the point estimate is only 1.16, and there is considerable (and statistically significant) heterogeneity among the estimates from the individual studies.

More uniformity of results is seen when duration of use is considered. Table B-21 shows results from 12 case-control studies that reported estimates of the relative risk of breast cancer in women under the age of 45 in relation to duration of use of oral contraceptives. In 2 of the studies, estimates from two age groups under 45 were combined, and in 2 others estimates from two categories of duration of use were combined, to provide more stable estimates for presentation in the table. The differences among the estimated relative risks can be explained on the basis of chance variation ($p = .21$), and a summary estimate of 1.42, with narrow confidence limits, was obtained by combining results from all studies in the table.

Although findings from a number of other case-control studies were not published in sufficient detail for inclusion in this table, most are broadly supportive of the results shown. Three reported increased relative risks in women under age 45, but did not present results in relation to duration of use (Fasal and Paffenbarger, 1979; Lee et al., 1987; Stanford et al., 1989). Two others reported increased relative risks in long-term users under age 45, but did not publish sufficient information for estimation of their confidence intervals (Lubin et al., 1982; Ravnihar et al., 1988). In four more studies, results were published only in relation to certain features of early use: two of these (Pike et al., 1983; Olsson et al., 1989) reported an increase in risk in relation to duration of use before age 25; three of the four (Paffenbarger et al., 1980; Harris et al., 1982; Olsson et al., 1989) reported an increased risk in relation to duration of use before a first full-term pregnancy. In addition, one of these studies (Olsson et al., 1989) reported that the relative risk of breast cancer in women who had ever used oral contraceptives increased with decreasing age at first use. Reanalysis of the data from these studies could well produce results similar to those in Table B-21.

Also supportive of the findings in Table B-21 are the recent results of one cohort study (Kay and Hannaford, 1988), which showed a strong trend of increasing risk related to duration of use in 30- to 34-year-old women (Table B-22). In the Nurses Health Study, Romieu and colleagues (1989) found a small increase in risk in women under age 45 who were using oral contraceptives when the cohort was established, but not in prior users. Although no significant increase in risk related to duration of use of oral contraceptives was found in 25- to 44-year-old women in the Oxford-Family Planning Association contraceptive cohort study (Vessey et al., 1989), rates are very slightly higher in users of more than 72 months' duration than in shorter-term users or nonusers.

Selective reporting of only positive results does not appear to be a likely explanation for the relative consistency of findings among studies. Only two case-control studies not shown in Table B-21, that have

TABLE B-22 Relative Risks of Breast Cancer in Women Under 45 Years of Age Who Have Ever Used Oral Contraceptives: Summary of Results from Cohort Studies

First Author (Date)	Age at Diagnosis	Years of Use	Cases per 1,000 Person-Years (No. of Cases)	Estimate of Relative Risk (Confidence Interval)[a]
Kay (1988)	<35	None	0.10(6)	1.00
		Ever	0.24(27)	2.38(0.98,5.76)
	30-34	None	0.12(4)	1.00
		<2	0.36(4)	3.00(0.85,10.69)
		2-3	0.40(6)	3.33(0.94,11.80)
		4-5	0.49(6)	4.08(1.15,14.46)
		6-7	0.26(2)	2.17(0.40,11.85)
		8-9	0.30(1)	2.50(0.28,22.37)
		<10	1.22(1)	10.17(1.14,90.99)
Romieu (1989)	30-34	None	0.52(9)	1.00
		Current	0.37(3)	0.71(0.19,2.60)
		Past	0.35(18)	0.67(0.30,1.40)
	35-39	None	0.83(43)	1.00
		Current	0.90(6)	1.00(0.43,2.35)
		Past	0.88(100)	1.05(0.74,1.51)
	40-44	None	1.12(104)	1.00
		Current	2.98(13)	2.66(1.53,4.63)
		Past	1.28(153)	1.14(0.89,1.46)
	<44	None	0.96(156)	1.00
		Current	1.15(22)	1.20[0.90,1.60]
		Past	0.95(271)	0.99[0.81,1.20]
Vessey (1989)	25-44	None	0.62(49)	1.00
		<2	0.56(9)	0.90[0.44,1.82]
		2-3	0.50(11)	0.81[0.42,1.55]
		4-5	0.61(16)	0.98[0.56,1.73]
		6-7	0.64(15)	1.03[0.57,1.85]
		8-9	0.65(12)	1.05[0.56,1.97]
		≥10	0.65(14)	1.05[0.58,1.89]

[a]Confidence interval of 95 percent used; [ ] = estimates from published data.

specifically addressed the issue of oral contraceptive use and risk of breast cancer in young women have not shown some evidence of an enhanced risk. One (Vessey et al., 1983) found relative risks of 1.01, 0.71, and 1.01 in users of more than eight years' duration among 16- to 35-year-old, 36- to 40-year-old, and 41- to 45-year-old women, respectively. The other study (La Vecchia et al., 1986) reported a relative risk of 0.87 in women under age 40 who had ever used oral contraceptives. No confidence intervals were given in the reports of either study. If the estimate of approximately a 40 percent increase in risk in young women who were long-term users is correct, a few studies could have failed to detect such a small enhancement in risk because of chance or insufficient statistical power.

Tables B-1 and B-2 illustrated that the relative risk of breast cancer in women of all ages combined who have ever used oral contraceptives is close to unity, with narrow confidence limits; it was also shown that there has been little overall increase in risk in long-term users (Table B-3 and B-4), or in women long after initial exposure (Table B-5 and B-6). Three possible interpretations of findings for young women are not incompatible with these overall results. One is that the proportion of cases under age 45 in most of the studies of women of all ages was relatively small, and the increased risk in young women may have contributed too little to the overall estimated value of the relative risk to elevate it appreciably above unity. A second possible interpretation is that women who have used oral contraceptives may tend to have their tumors diagnosed earlier than do nonusers, due to more screening or breast self-examination (screening bias). A third possibility is that oral contraceptives stimulate growth of breast carcinomas, so that women who are destined to develop them tend to do so at an earlier age (growth stimulation). The latter two explanations would eventually result in an observed reduction in risk in women at some time beyond age 45, and no overall alteration of risk.

Table B-23 shows relative risks in long-term users for women in various age groups above and below 45 years. Three of the studies (Paul et al., 1986; McPherson et al., 1987; Vessey et al., 1989) are supportive of either of the latter two possibilities given above, in that relative risks are greater than 1.0 in young women, and under 1.0 in older women. The three other studies shown in the table, however, do not show this variation in relative risks by age.

Other evidence that oral contraceptives are associated with earlier diagnosis or tumor growth stimulation would be a rise, and then a fall, in relative risk with duration of use in current users (as a surrogate for risk in relation to time from initial exposure in women who continue to take the pill). The first three studies shown in Table B-24 reported relative risks by duration of use in women who were last exposed within the previous year. As shown in column 1 of the table, two of these studies (Rosenberg et al., 1984; CASH, 1986) showed some increase and then a fall in relative risk in relation to duration of use in current users, but the WHO (1990) study did not. One might also expect to see a decline in risk with time since last exposure in women in those duration-of-use categories in which an increase in risk in current users was observed. This trend is apparent only in the WHO study.

TABLE B-23   Relative Risks of Breast Cancer in Long-term Users of Oral Contraceptives by Age at Diagnosis

First Author (Date)[a]	Duration of Use	Age at Diagnosis	Relative Risk
Vessey (1983)	≥8 years	16-35	1.01
		36-40	0.71
		41-45	1.01
		46-50	1.07
Rosenberg (1984)	≥5 years	20-29	0.8
		30-39	1.3
		40-49	0.9
		50-59	1.7
Paul (1986)	≥10 years	25-34	4.6
		35-44	0.84
		45-54	0.96
McPherson (1987)	≥12 years	<45	1.78
		≥45	0.84
Ravnihar (1988)	≥7 years	25-34	1.26
		35-44	2.63
		45-54	2.15
Vessey (1989)	>10 years	25-44	1.05
		≥45	0.48

[a]All studies in the table are case-control designs except Vessey, which is a cohort design.

A consideration of the histological features of breast tumors that have developed in users of oral contraceptives provides some suggestion that these products may stimulate tumor growth. Romieu and colleagues (1989) found tumors in users to be larger and more often metastatic at diagnosis than those in nonusers (although this has not been observed by others, as indicated in the next section); Kay and Hannaford (1988) found that tumors in women under age 35 were of a somewhat higher grade in users than nonusers; and Stanford and coworkers (1989) observed, in women in a screening program, a relative risk for in situ tumors of 0.57 in relation to more than five years of oral contraceptive use, but relative risks of 1.54 and 1.37 for small and large invasive tumors, respectively.

Screening Bias

If an observed association between oral contraceptives and breast cancer is a result of users being diagnosed because of more intensive

TABLE B-24   Relative Risk of Breast Cancer by Duration of Use and Time Since Last Use of Oral Contraceptives

First Author (Date)	Years of Use	Years Since Last Use					
		<1	1-4	5-9	10-14	≥10	≥15
Rosenberg	<1	0	1.0	1.1	0.7		1.2
(1984)	1-4	0.7	0.8	1.0	1.1		0.8
	5-9	1.4	0.9	1.3		1.7	
	≥10	0.9	0.9	0.6		1.1	

		<1	1-4	5-9	10-14	≥15
CASH[a] (1986)	<1	1.0	1.2	1.0	0.8	1.0
	1-2	1.5	1.0	1.4[b]	0.9	0.9
	3-5	1.5	1.6[b]	1.1	1.0	0.8
	6-9	1.1	1.2	1.3	1.1	0.1[b]
	10-14	1.0	1.1	1.3	1.0	
	≥15	0.5	1.1	0.2[b]		

		<5	5-9	10-14	≥15
Miller (1989)	>5	2.7	1.7	1.7	6.0

		3	6	9	12
U.K. National	1-4	1.01	1.29	1.08	0.95
Case-Control	5-8	1.42	1.47	1.63	1.23
Study Group	>8	2.22	3.10		
(1989)[d]					

		<1/4	1/4-3	4-9	>10
WHO[c]	<1	2.07	1.23	1.23	1.01
(1990)	1-2	1.41	1.63	1.10	0.88
	3-8	1.19	1.53	1.20	0.60
	>8	2.16	1.38	1.12	0.76

[a]CASH = Cancer and Steroid Hormone Study.
[b]Ninety-five percent confidence interval of estimate excludes 1.0.
[c]WHO = World Health Organization.
[d]Calculated by eliminating and controlling for use before years since last use shown.

screening (or breast self-examination), then one would expect tumors in users, and perhaps especially in long-term and recent users, to be smaller and more locally confined than tumors in nonusers. The U.K. National Case-Control Study Group (1989), Kay and Hannaford (1988), and Miller and coworkers (1989) all found trends of increasing relative risk in young women with duration of use (Tables B-21 and B-22), but none of these three studies found convincing evidence for a screening bias. Only small differences between users and nonusers in the size of tumors and in the extent of the disease at diagnosis were observed by the U.K. group and by the Miller team. In addition, in the former study, breast self-examination was practiced with equal frequency by users and nonusers, although a higher proportion of exposed than unexposed women had had a breast examination in the past year. The results of Kay and Hannaford (1988) could not be explained by differential screening in users because few women (6 percent of users and 4 percent of nonusers) had their tumor diagnosed as a result of screening for breast cancer.

In the WHO (1990) study risk was particularly enhanced in relation to use in low-risk countries, and in relation to long-term and recent use. Yet, individuals characterized by such use were not more likely than other users or nonusers to have smaller tumors or more localized disease at diagnosis. A small increase in risk in women who had used oral contraceptives for more than three years before age 25 was also observed in that study and such users did tend to have small tumors, but users of shorter duration, with an equally high relative risk, did not. The small increase in relative risk in relation to use before a woman's first live birth that was observed in the WHO study was found to be confined to women who had had an aborted pregnancy or stillbirth prior to their first live birth. In those cases the tumors tended to be smaller than the tumors in other women, suggesting the possibility of enhanced surveillance for breast cancer in this small group.

On balance, it appears unlikely that the major positive finding from these studies (and by inference from other studies as well) can be explained by enhanced screening in users of oral contraceptives.

Risk in Relation to Use of Oral Contraceptives Near the Age of Menopause

Women who go through the menopause late in life are at higher risk for breast cancer than women with an early natural or artificial menopause. If use of oral contraceptives late in a woman's potentially reproductive years were to simulate endocrinologically a late menopause, one would expect such use to increase a woman's risk of breast cancer. This possibility has not been adequately investigated, but results of analyses relevant to this question are summarized in Table B-25. The findings are equivocal. Three studies show increased relative risks in users over age 45 (Vessey et al., 1979; Yuan et al., 1988) or over age 50 (Jick et al., 1980), but this was not observed by Rosenberg and colleagues (1984). In addition, although use of oral contraceptives

TABLE B-25   Relative Risks of Breast Cancer in Women Who Used
Combined Oral Contraceptives Near the Age of Menopause

First Author (Date)	Definition of Exposure	Age or Years of Use	Relative Risk	Confidence Interval (95%)
Vessey (1979)	Use in past year	41-45 years old	0.85	Not given
		46-50 years old	2.57	Not given
Jick (1980)	Current use	41-45 years old	0.8	0.1,4.6
		46-50 years old	4.0	1.8,9.0
		51-55 years old	15.5	5.2,46
Rosenberg (1984)	Use in past year	40-49 years old	0.9	0.4,1.9
		50-59 years old	1.0	0.1,1.7
Yuan (1988)	Any use after age 45	Any use	4.00	1.15,16.59
Stanford (1989)	Premenopausal years of use after age 40	<2 years	0.95	Includes 1.0
		2-3 years	1.46	Includes 1.0
		4-5 years	1.03	Includes 1.0
		6-7 years	1.18	Includes 1.0
		≥8 years	1.05	Includes 1.0
	Postmenopausal years of use after age 40	<2 years	0.76	Includes 1.0
		2-3 years	0.51	Includes 1.0
		4-5 years	0.97	Includes 1.0
		6-7 years	1.49	Includes 1.0
		≥8 years	1.00	Includes 1.0
Romieu (1989)	Use up to 2 years before diagnosis	40-44 years old	2.66	1.53,4.63
		45-49 years old	1.63	0.81,3.27
		50-54 years old	1.13	0.28,4.45

up to two years prior to diagnosis was associated with an elevated risk
in three age groups above 39 years in the Nurses Health Study (Romieu
et al., 1989), the relative risks were lower in 50- to 54-year-old women
than in younger women. There is a suggestion of an increase in risk in
users of from six to seven years after age 40 in postmenopausal women in the study of Stanford and colleagues (1989), but not in users of
eight or more years' duration. Data from other studies should be analyzed to address this issue further, with particular emphasis on use that
extends into the sixth decade of life.

Individual Formulations and Constituents of Oral Contraceptives

In 1983, Pike and coworkers reported that risk of breast cancer was
particularly increased in association with use before age 25 of oral
contraceptives with a high progestin potency, as determined by the

delay of menses test. This result may have been an artifact, however, that arose from the erroneous classification of one particular product as being of high potency (Armstrong, 1986). For purposes of comparison, results from the CASH Study (Stadel et al., 1985) were presented using the same classification scheme, and relative risks in users of products classified as of high progestin potency were not found to be significantly increased. Relative risks associated with four categories of duration, the longest being greater than 74 months, varied from 1.1 to 1.3 but did not increase with length of exposure. Miller and colleagues (1986) also did not confirm the findings of the Pike study. Relative risks of 1.0 (CI = 0.5,2.2) and 1.1 (CI = 0.4,3.0) were observed in users of two "high progestin potency" pills (Ovral and Ovulen l, respectively).

In 1987, McPherson and coworkers reported an increase in risk in relation to duration of use before a woman's first full-term pregnancy with oral contraceptives that contain the estrogen ethinyl estradiol, but not in relation to similar use of preparations containing mestranol. However, this result was not confirmed by Schlesselman and coworkers (1987) or Vessey and colleagues (1989).

Three groups of investigators have reported relative risks in relation to use at any time of preparations containing ethinyl estradiol and mestranol. As shown in Table B-26, no study shows a stronger association with breast cancer for one type of estrogen than the other. Table B-27 similarly shows that no specific type of progestin has been implicated as being particularly associated with breast cancer risk. It should be noted that all of the progestins shown in the table except megestrol acetate are derivatives of 19-nor-testosterone. Formulations containing 17-α-hyroxyprogesterone derivatives (i.e., medroxyprogesterone acetate and chlormadinone) were shown to cause mammary tumors in beagle dogs, and were subsequently withdrawn from the market in many countries, including the United States. These products are in use in some countries of the world and were investigated in the WHO (1990) study. Analyses to assess the relative risk of breast cancer in users of such products are in progress, but results are not yet available.

Finally, results from three studies that estimated relative risks of breast cancer in relation to specific pill types are summarized in Table B-28. No single formulation is consistently related to breast cancer across all three studies. Also, relative risks do not appear to be uniformly higher for the higher dose products (shown near the top of each section of the table) than for the lower dose pills. In support of these observations, Ravnihar and colleagues (1988) and Vessey and coworkers (1989) found no appreciable differences in the distribu-

TABLE B-26 Associations Between Breast Cancer and Dosages of Mestranol and Ethinyl Estradiol in Oral Contraceptives

First Author (Date)	Dosage	Measure of Association	Mestranol	Ethinyl Estradiol
CASH[a] (1986)	<1.0 mg-mo[b]	Relative	0.8(0.7,1.1)	1.1(0.8,1.4)
	1.0-2.9 mg-mo	risk	1.0(0.8,1.2)	0.9(0.7,1.2)
	3.0-4.9 mg-mo		1.1(0.9,1.4)	1.3(0.9,1.9)
	≥5.0 mg-mo		1.1(0.9,1.3)	0.8(0.5,1.2)
	Any use		1.0(0.9,1.1)	1.0(0.8,1.2)
U.K. National	<50/<100 micrograms[c]	Relative	1.08	1.04
Case-Control	≥50/≥100 micrograms[e]	risk[a,d]	1.03	1.12
Study Group (1989)	Any strength		1.09	1.08
Vessey (1989)	30/50 micrograms[f]	Mean	1.02	1.04
	50/100 micrograms[g]	months used	0.82	0.86
	100/___ micrograms[h]	in cases/	N.a.	0.60
	Any strength	mean months		
		in controls	0.95	0.89

N.a. = Not applicable.
[a]CASH = Cancer and Steroid Hormone Study.
[b]mg-mo = Milligram - months of use.
[c]<50 Micrograms ethinyl estradiol or <100 micrograms mestranol.
[d]Estimated from published report by calculating mean relative risks weighted by woman-months of use.
[e]≥50 Micrograms ethinyl estradiol or ≥100 micrograms mestranol.
[f]30 Micrograms ethinyl estradiol or 50 micrograms mestranol.
[g]50 Micrograms ethinyl estradiol or 100 micrograms mestranol.
[h]100 Micrograms ethinyl estradiol.

TABLE B-27 Associations Reported in Two Studies Between Breast Cancer and Types of Progestins in Oral Contraceptives

Progestin	CASH[a] (1986)	Vessey[b] (1989)
Ethynodiol diacetate[c]	1.1(0.9,1.4)	0.7
Norethindrone	1.1(1.0,1.3)	1.1
Norethindrone acetate[c]	1.1(0.7,1.6)	1.3
Norethynodrel	0.8(0.6,0.9)	
Norgestrel (LorDL)	1.0(0.8,1.3)	1.0
Lynoestrenol[c]		0.9
Megestrol acetate		0.9

[a]CASH = Cancer and Steroid Hormone Study. Relative risks in women who only took oral contraceptives with the specific progestin shown. Parentheses indicated 95 percent confidence intervals.
[b]Ratios of mean months of use in cases to mean months of use in controls.
[c]Metabolized to norethindrone (Norethisterone).

TABLE B-28   Relative Risks of Breast Cancer in Women Who Have Ever Used Specific Types of Oral Contraceptives

Micrograms of Mestranol	Progestin Type	Milligrams	CASH (1986)[a]	Miller (1989)[b]	U.K. Study[c] (1989)
100	Ethynodiol diacetate	1.0	1.1(0.9,1.4)	1.1(0.4,2.9)	0.95
100	Norethynodrel	2.5	0.7(0.5,0.9)	2.6(0.6,11)	
100	Norethisterone	2.0	1.3(1.0,1.7)	1.9(0.5,7.1)	1.18
80	Norethisterone	1.0	1.0(0.8,1.3)	0.7(0.2,2.6)	
75	Lynestrenol	2.5			0.87
75	Norethynodrel	5.0	0.8(0.5,1.3)		
60	Norethisterone	10.0	0.6(0.3,1.3)		
50	Norethisterone	1.0	1.2(0.9,1.5)	3.3(1.5,7.1)	1.10
Micrograms of Estradiol					
50	Ethynodiol diacetate	1.0	1.0(0.6,1.6)	1.0(0.3,3.6)	1.26
50	Lynestrenol	2.5			1.13
50	Megestrol acetate	4.0			0.96
50	Norethisterone acetate	4.0			1.36
50	Norethisterone acetate	3.0			1.09
50	Norethisterone acetate	2.5			1.21
50	Norethisterone acetate	1.0	1.6(0.9,2.8)	1.0(0.2,5.4)	1.11
50	Norgestrel	0.5	0.9(0.7,1.2)	1.8(1.0,3.3)	1.05[d]
35	Norethisterone	0.5	0.8(0.5,1.2)		1.18
32	Levonorgestrel	0.09			0.83
30	Norgestrel	0.30	0.7(0.4,1.3)	0.8(0.3,2.1)	
30	Levonorgestrel	0.25			1.00
30	Levonorgestrel	0.15			1.08
20	Norethisterone acetate	1.0			1.36

[a]CASH = Cancer and Steroid Hormone Study; ( ) = confidence interval of 95 percent.
[b]( ) = confidence interval of 95 percent.
[c]U.K. Study = U.K. National Case-Control Study Group.
[d]Relative risk was estimated by calculating the mean of the relative risks for two different products that contain 0.25 milligrams Levonorgestrel, weighted by woman-months of use.

tions of cases and controls by type of pill used. In addition, Vessey and colleagues found no difference in the distributions of person-years of exposure of cases and controls to specific formulations.

CONCLUSIONS, INTERPRETATIONS, AND
RECOMMENDATIONS FOR FURTHER RESEARCH

Oral contraceptives, as they have been used to date, have caused little or no overall increase in the risk of breast cancer in women in developed countries. Risks in women of all ages combined have not been appreciably enhanced by more than a decade of exposure or after a potential latent period of up to two decades.

Limited information from developing countries, where rates of breast cancer are much lower than in the developed countries where most studies of oral contraceptives and breast cancer have been conducted, suggests that oral contraceptive use may moderately enhance risk in women in low-risk populations. A possible mechanism for this increase is the stimulation of proliferative activity in the stem cells of the lobular epithelium. Such stimulation may not occur to a measurable extent in high-risk populations of women, whose lobular epithelia may already be maximally stimulated by other (unknown) factors that put these women at high risk. Further studies in low-risk populations are warranted.

Oral contraceptives do not appear to have a differential impact on risk in women with and without such risk factors for breast cancer as high socioeconomic status, nulliparity, low parity, a late first full-term pregnancy (or live birth), or a family history of breast cancer. Compared to risks of breast cancer among countries, which may differ by a factor of 10, the risks in women with and without each of these risk factors differ by a factor of only about 2 or 3. The potential for the lobular epithelium of the breast of women without these risk factors to be further stimulated by oral contraceptives, compared with this potential in women with these factors, may thus be smaller than the differential potential for lobular stimulation in women in low- and high-risk populations. (It may also be too small to measure by epidemiological means.) Further study of the influence of oral contraceptives in women with and without the generally recognized risk factors for breast cancer should not receive high priority.

Limited information suggests that oral contraceptives (whether used before or after a benign lesion) may enhance the risk of breast cancer in young women with a prior history of benign breast disease but not in older women with such a history. Because the benign lesions in younger women are more likely than the benign lesions in older women to be fibroadenomas, further study of this issue should include young women in particular. It should also include a slide review to characterize the prior benign lesion histologically. In women of all ages combined, the use of oral contraceptives after benign lesions has not been shown to enhance risk. The suggested study in young women should distinguish between use before and after the prior benign condition.

Multiple studies of varying types have not consistently shown women who used oral contraceptives before the birth of their first child, or before the age of 25 years, to be at increased risk of breast cancer. Results among studies are more consistent for an increase in risk in women under the age of 45 who were long-term users of oral contraceptives (regardless of whether use occurred before or after a first birth or a particular age). Such users would, of course, tend to have been young at their initial use.

This observed increase in risk is not likely to be due to differential screening for breast cancer in oral contraceptive users. There is suggestive but inconsistent evidence that it could be a result of the pill stimulating growth in preexisting tumors. Alternatively, oral contraceptives, when used early in life, could be causing a small absolute increase in risk in young women. It is of extreme importance to determine which of these two possible biological mechanisms may be operating. If it is the former, then oral contraceptives are not causing any new breast cancers; if it is the latter, they are, and this could theoretically continue and become even more of a problem with the aging of the cohort of women who have been exposed early in life. Rigorous epidemiological studies should therefore be conducted to continue monitoring for any enhanced risk of breast cancer among women in birth cohorts exposed at a young age to prolonged use of oral contraceptives. Such studies should not be confined to women below a specific arbitrary age. They should include a pathological component to measure indices of proliferative activity and determine the likely cells of origin of the tumors (whether ductal or lobular). The analyses of both the histologic and epidemiological data should be planned to provide evidence for or against the two above-mentioned biological mechanisms.

Studies of survival in women with breast cancer would also be of value. If oral contraceptive users have more favorable survival than nonusers, this pattern would be evidence for a screening bias (or suggest that breast tumors that develop in response to oral contraceptives are less aggressive than other breast tumors). If survival is less favorable in users than in nonusers, this pattern would be evidence that oral contraceptives stimulate tumor growth (or suggest that breast tumors that develop in response to oral contraceptives are more aggressive than other breast tumors).

Limited evidence suggests that use of oral contraceptives near the time of menopause may increase a woman's risk of breast cancer. A possible mechanism for this is endocrinologic simulation of a delayed menopause by the exogenous estrogens and progestins. Further investigation of this issue is also warranted, perhaps most efficiently by reanalysis of data from existing studies, to estimate relative risks in relation to duration of use in women in their late 40s and 50s.

No difference in possible associations with breast cancer has been observed between oral contraceptive formulations that contain mestranol and those that contain ethinyl estradiol. This finding is not surprising because the former is metabolized to the latter and the active estrogen is thus the same in both types of preparations. The progestins in almost all contraceptives that have been considered in studies of breast cancer to date are derivatives of 19-nor-testosterone. None have consistently been shown to be more strongly associated with breast cancer than others. Results of studies of oral contraceptives that contain 17-α-hydroxyprogesterone derivatives have not been published. Recent studies from New Zealand (Paul et al., 1989) and Costa Rica (Lee et al., 1987) have shown a possible increase in risk of breast cancer in some categories of users of the long-acting progestational agent depot-medroxyprogesterone acetate (DMPA), which is a 17-α-hydroxyprogesterone derivative.

Results from the WHO (1990) study of both DMPA and oral contraceptives that contain chlormadinone are pending. In view of the existing findings on DMPA and reports of these progestational agents causing breast cancer in beagle dogs, additional studies of breast cancer in relation to products with these types of progestins may be warranted, particularly if the results from the WHO study are not reassuring.

ACKNOWLEDGMENTS

The statistical analyses reported in this appendix were performed by Elizabeth A. Noonan. The author thanks James Schlesselman and David Skegg for their helpful comments.

REFERENCES

Armstrong, B. K. 1986. Oral contraceptives and breast cancer (letter). Lancet 1:552.
Brinton, L. A., R. Hoover, M. Szklo, and J. F. Fraumeni, Jr. 1982. Oral contraceptives and breast cancer. International Journal of Epidemiology 11:316-322.
(CASH) Cancer and Steroid Hormone Study of the Centers for Disease Control and the National Institute of Child Health and Human Development. 1986. Oral contraceptive use and the risk of breast cancer. New England Journal of Medicine 315:405-411.
Clavel, F., M. Le, and A. LaPlanche. 1981. Breast cancer and use of antihypertensive

drugs and oral contraceptives: Results of a case-control study. Bulletin du Cancer 68:449-455.

Ellery, C., R. MacLennan, G. Berry, and R. P. Shearman. 1986. A case-control study of breast cancer in relation to the use of steroid contraceptive agents. Medical Journal of Australia 144:173-176.

Fasal, E., and R. S. Paffenbarger, Jr. 1979. Oral contraceptives as related to cancer and benign lesions of the breast. Journal of the National Cancer Institute 55:767-773.

Harris, N. V., N. S. Weiss, A. M. Francis, and L. Polissar. 1982. Breast cancer in relation to patterns of oral contraceptive use. American Journal of Epidemiology 116:643-651.

Henderson, B. E., D. Powell, I. Rosario, C. Keys, R. Hanish, M. Young, J. Casagrande, V. Gerkins, and M. C. Pike. 1974. An epidemiologic study of breast cancer. Journal of the National Cancer Institute 53:609-614.

Hennekens, C. H., F. E. Speizer, R. J. Lipnick, B. Roser, C. Bain, C. Belanger, M. J. Stampfer, W. Willet, and R. Peto. 1984. A case-control study of oral contraceptives use and breast cancer. Journal of the National Cancer Institute 72:39-42.

Janerich, D. T., A. P. Polednak, D. M. Glebatis, and C. E. Lawrence. 1983. Breast cancer and oral contraceptive use: A case-control study. Journal of Chronic Disease 36:639-646.

Jick, H., A. M. Walker, R. N. Watkins, D. C. D'Ewart, J. R. Hunter, A. Danford, S. Madsen, B. J. Dian, and K. J. Rothman. 1980. Oral contraceptives and breast cancer. American Journal of Epidemiology 112:577-585.

Jick, S. S., A. M. Walker, A. Stergachis, and H. Jick. 1989. Oral contraceptives and breast cancer. British Journal of Cancer 59:618-621.

Kay, C. R., and P. C. Hannaford. 1988. Breast cancer and the pill—A further report from the Royal College of General Practitioners' Oral Contraception Study. British Journal of Cancer 58:675-680.

Kelsey, J. L., T. R. Holford, C. White, E. S. Mayer, S. E. Kilty, and R. M. Acheson. 1978. Oral contraceptives and breast disease: An epidemiological study. American Journal of Epidemiology 107:236-244.

Kelsey, J. L., D. B. Fischer, T. R. Holford, V. A. LiVolsi, E. D. Mostow, I. S. Goldenberg, and C. White. 1981. Exogeneous estrogens and other factors in the epidemiology of breast cancer. Journal of the National Cancer Institute 67:327-333.

La Vecchia, C., A. Decarli, M. Fasoli, S. Franceschi, A. Gentile, E. Negri, F. Parazzini, and G. Tognoni. 1986. Oral contraceptives and cancers of the breast and of the female genital tract. Interim results from a case-control study. British Journal of Cancer 54:311-317.

Lee, N. C., L. Rosero-Bixby, M. W. Oberle, C. Grimaldo, A. S. Whatley, and E. Z. Rovira. 1987. A case-control study of breast cancer and hormonal contraception in Costa Rica. Journal of the National Cancer Institute 79:1247-1254.

Lees, A. W., P. E. Burns, and M. Grace. 1978. Oral contraceptives and breast disease in premenopausal northern Albertan women. International Journal of Cancer 22:700-707.

Lipnick, R. J., J. E. Buring, C. H. Hennekens, B. Rosner, W. Willet, C. Bain, M. J. Stampfer, G. A. Colditz, R. Peto, and F. E. Speizer. 1986. Oral contraceptives and breast cancer. Journal of the American Medical Association 255:58-61.

Lubin, J. H., P. E. Burns, W. J. Blot, A. W. Lees, C. May, L. E. Morris, and J. F. Fraumeni, Jr. 1982. Risk factors for breast cancer in women in northern Alberta, Canada, as related to age at diagnosis. Journal of the National Cancer Institute 68:211-217.

Lund, E., O. Meirik, H. Adami, R. Bergstrom, T. Christoffersen, and P. Bergsjo. 1989. Oral contraceptive use and premenopausal breast cancer in Sweden and Norway:

Possible effects of different pattern of use. International Journal of Epidemiology 18:527-532.

McPherson, K., P. A. Coope, and M. P. Vessey. 1986. Early oral contraceptive use and breast cancer: Theoretical effects of latency. Journal of Epidemiology and Community Health 40:289-294.

McPherson, K., M. P. Vessey, A. Neil, R. Doll, L. Jones, and M. Roberts. 1987. Early oral contraceptive use and breast cancer: Results of another case-control study. British Journal of Cancer 56:653-660.

Meirik, O., E. Lund, H. O. Adami, R. Bergstrom, T. Christofferson, and P. Bergsjo, 1986. Oral contraceptive use and breast cancer in young women. A joint national case-control study in Sweden and Norway. Lancet 2:650-654.

Meirik, O., T. M. M. Farley, E. Lund, H. O. Adami, T. Christofferson, and P. Bergsjo. 1989. Breast cancer and oral contraceptives: Patterns of risk among parous and nulliparous women—further analysis of the Swedish-Norwegan material. Contraception 39:471-475.

Miller, D. R., L. Rosenberg, D. W. Kaufman, D. Schottenfeld, P. D. Stolley, and S. Shapiro. 1986. Breast cancer risk in relation to early oral contraceptive use. Obstetrics and Gynecology 68:863-868.

Miller, D. R., L. Rosenberg, D. W. Kaufman, P. Stolley, M. E. Warshauer, and S. Shapiro. 1989. Breast cancer before age 45 and oral contraceptive use: New findings. American Journal of Epidemiology 129:269-280.

Mills, P. K., W. L. Beeson, R. L. Phillips, and G. E. Fraser. 1989. Prospective study of exogenous hormone use and breast cancer in Seventh-Day Adventists. Cancer 64:591-597.

Olsson, H., T. R. Moller, and J. Ranstam. 1989. Early oral contraceptive use and breast cancer among premenopausal women: Final report from a study in southern Sweden. Journal of the National Cancer Institute 81:1000-1004.

Paffenbarger, R. S., E. Fasal, M. E. Simmons, and J. B. Kampert. 1977. Cancer risk as related to use of oral contraceptives during fertile years. Cancer 39:1887-1891.

Paffenbarger, R. S., J. B. Kampert, and H. G. Chang. 1980. Characteristics that predict risk of breast cancer before and after the menopause. American Journal of Epidemiology 112:258-268.

Paul, C., D. C. G. Skegg, G. F. S. Spears, and J. M. Kaldor. 1986. Oral contraceptives and breast cancer: A national study. British Medical Journal 293:723-726.

Paul, C., D. C. G. Skegg, and G. F. S. Spears. 1989. Depot medroxyprogesterone (Depo-Provera) and risk of breast cancer. British Medical Journal 299:759-762.

Paul, C., D. C. G. Skegg, and G. F. S. Spears. 1990. Oral contraception and breast cancer in New Zealand. Pp. 85-94 in Oral Contraceptives and Breast Cancer, R. D. Mann, ed. Park Ridge, N.J.: The Parthenon Publishing Group.

Pike, M. C., B. E. Henderson, J. T. Casagrande, I. Rosario, and G. E. Gray. 1981. Oral contraceptive use and early abortion as risk factors for breast cancer in young women. British Journal of Cancer 43:72-76.

Pike, M. C., B. E. Henderson, M. D. Krailo, A. Duke, and S. Roy. 1983. Breast cancer in young women and use of oral contraceptives: Possible modifying effect of formulation and age at use. Lancet 2:926-930.

Prentice, R. L., and D. B. Thomas. 1986. On the epidemiology of oral contraceptives and disease. Advances in Cancer Research 49:285-401.

Ravnihar, B., D. G. Seigel, and J. Lindtner. 1979. An epidemiologic study of breast cancer and benign breast neoplasia in relation to the oral contraceptive and estrogen use. European Journal of Cancer 15:395-405.

Ravnihar, B., M. Primic Zakelj, K. Kosmelj, and J. Stare. 1988. A case-control study of breast cancer in relation to oral contraceptive use in Slovenia. Neoplasma 35:109-120.

Romieu, I., W. C. Willett, G. A. Colditz, M. J. Stampfer, B. Rosner, C. H. Hennekens, and F. E. Speizer. 1989. Prospective study of oral contraceptive use and risk of breast cancer in women. Journal of the National Cancer Institute 81:1313-1321.

Rosenberg, L., D. R. Miller, D. W. Kaufman, S. P. Helmrich, P. D. Stolley, D. Schottenfeld, and S. Shapiro. 1984. Breast cancer and oral contraceptive use. American Journal of Epidemiology 119:167-176.

Sartwell, P. E., F. G. Arthes, and J. A. Tonascia. 1977. Exogeneous hormones, reproductive history and breast cancer. Journal of the National Cancer Institute 59:1589-1592.

Schlesselman, J. J., B. V. Stadel, P. Murray, and S. Lai. 1987. Breast cancer risk in relation to type of estrogen contained in oral contraceptives. Contraception 36:595-613.

Schlesselman, J. J., B. V. Stadel, P. Murray, and S. Lai. 1988. Breast cancer in relation to early use of oral contraceptives: No evidence of latent effect. Journal of the American Medical Association 259:1828-1833.

Stadel, B. V., and J. J. Schlesselman. 1986. Oral contraceptive use and the risk of breast cancer in women with a "prior" history of benign breast disease. American Journal of Epidemiology 123:373-382.

Stadel, B. V., G. L. Rubin, L. A. Webster, J. J. Schlesselman, and P. A. Wingo. 1985. Oral contraceptives and breast cancer in young women. Lancet 2:970-973.

Stadel, B. V., J. J. Schlesselman, and P. A. Murray. 1989. Oral contraceptives and breast cancer. Lancet 1:1257-1258.

Stalsberg, H., D. B. Thomas, E. A. Noonan, and the WHO Collaborative Study of Neoplasia and Steroid Contraceptives. 1989. Histologic types of breast carcinoma in relation to international variation and breast cancer risk factors. International Journal of Cancer 44:399-409.

Stanford, J. L., L. A. Brinton, and R. N. Hoover. 1989. Oral contraceptives and breast cancer: Results from an expanded case-control study. British Journal of Cancer 60:375-381.

Talamini, R., C. La Vecchia, S. Franceschi, F. Colombo, A. Decarli, E. Grattoni, E. Grigoletto, and G. Tognoni. 1985. Reproductive and hormonal factors and breast cancer in a northern Italian population. International Journal of Epidemiology 14:70-74.

Thomas, D. B. 1989. The breast. Pp. 38-68 in Safety Requirements for Contraceptive Steroids, F. Michal, ed. Cambridge: Cambridge University Press.

Trapido, E. J. 1981. A prospective cohort study of oral contraceptives and breast cancer. Journal of the National Cancer Institute 67:1011-1015.

U.K. National Case-Control Study Group. 1989. Oral contraceptive use and breast cancer risk in young women. Lancet 1:973-982.

Vessey, M. P., R. Doll, K. Jones, K. McPherson, and D. Yeates. 1979. An epidemiological study of oral contraceptives and breast cancer. British Medical Journal 1:1755-1778.

Vessey, M. P., K. McPherson, and R. Doll. 1981. Breast cancer and oral contraceptives: Findings in Oxford-Family Planning Association Contraceptive Study. British Medical Journal 282:2093-2094.

Vessey, M. P., K. McPherson, D. Yeates, and R. Doll. 1982. Oral contraceptive use and abortion before first term pregnancy in relation to breast cancer risk. British Journal of Cancer 45:327-331.

Vessey, M., J. Baron, R. Doll, K. McPherson, and D. Yeates. 1983. Oral contraceptives and breast cancer: Final report of an epidemiological study. British Journal of Cancer 47:455-462.

Vessey, M. P., K. McPherson, L. Villard-Mackintosh, and D. Yeates. 1989. Oral contraceptives and breast cancer: Latest findings in a large cohort study. British Journal of Cancer 59:613-617.

(WHO) World Health Organization Collaborative Study of Neoplasia and Steroid Contraceptives. 1990. Breast cancer and combined oral contraceptives: Results from a multinational study. British Journal of Cancer 61:110-119.

Yuan, J., M. Yu, R. K. Ross, Y. T. Gao, and B. E. Henderson. 1988. Risk factors for breast concer in Chinese women in Shanghai. Cancer Research 48:1949-1953.

C

The Evolving Formulations of Oral Contraceptives

Over the past 25 years, populations of oral contraceptive users have progressed through a continuum of formulations ranging from doses as high as 150 micrograms (µg) of estrogen and 10 milligrams (mg) of progestin to the current formulations, which use 30 to 40 µg of estrogen and 1.5 mg or less of progestin. Following a recommendation by its Fertility and Maternal Health Drugs Advisory Committee, the Food and Drug Administration (FDA) recently ordered the removal from the market of all oral contraceptives with estrogen contents greater than 50 µg. As a result of this decision, there are currently 17 different formulations of the pill available in the United States, which are marketed under 29 brand names (see Tables C-1, C-2, and C-3). Different regimens (i.e., 21- and 28-day) of the same formulation are considered to be one brand.

The changing formulations also brought a change in the prescribing preferences and practices of physicians. Today, the most commonly prescribed oral contraceptive for new users in the United States is Ortho 7/7/7, which combines 35 µg of ethinyl estradiol with 0.5 to 1 mg of norethindrone (Contraceptive Technology Update, 1989). Four other triphasics are also available (Table C-3). Triphasic formulations are generally thought to be an improvement over the monophasic

Appendix C is a product of the IOM Committee on the Relationship Between Oral Contraceptives and Breast Cancer.

TABLE C-1 Summary of Estrogen and Progestin Contents of Oral Contraceptives Available in the United States, 20- to 35-μg Formulations

Brand Name[a]	Estrogen per Tablet (μg)	Total Estrogen (μg)	Progestin Type	Progestin per Tablet (mg)	Total Progestin (mg)	Approximate Equivalents[b] (mg)
Loestrin 1/20	20	420	Norethindrone acetate	1.0	21.0	21.0
Loestrin 1.5/30	30	630	Norethindrone acetate	1.5	31.5	31.5
LoOvral[c]	30	630	Levonorgestrel	0.15	3.15	31.5-63.0
Levlen						
Nordette						
Ovcon 35	35	735	Norethindrone	0.4	8.4	8.4
Brevicon	35	735	Norethindrone	0.5	10.5	10.5
Genora 0.5/35						
Modicon						
Genora 1/35	35	735	Norethindrone	1.0	21.0	21.0
Norcept-E 1/35						
Norethin 1/35E						
Norinyl 1+35						
Ortho-Novum 1/35						
Demulen 1/35	32	735	Ethinodiol diacetate	1.0	21.0	21.0

[a]Regimens of both 21 and 28 days are listed as the same formulation.
[b]Based on estimates of approximate progestin potencies (reviewed by Dorflinger, 1985).
[c]Also contains the inactive enantiomer dextronorgestrel.

formulations in that the total steroid dose can be reduced without compromising effectiveness in preventing pregnancy or cycle control. It should be noted, however, that the triphasic formulations containing norethindrone are actually slightly higher in total hormone dose than the two lowest-dose monophasic formulations that contain the same two hormones (Ovcon 35, and Brevicon/Modicon/ Genora 0.5/35; Tables C-1 and C-3).

Over the next five years, a number of new oral contraceptive formulations are likely to become available in the American market. Several of these (e.g., Cilest, Marvelon, and Femodene; see Table C-4) are already marketed in a number of countries worldwide, including many European countries. Cilest, which will be marketed as Ortho-Cyclen in the United States, was recently approved by the FDA. These products are all low-estrogen formulations—30 or 35 μg of ethinyl estradiol. They contain new 19-nortestosterone progestins, which are

TABLE C-2 Summary of Estrogen and Progestin Contents of Oral Contraceptives Available in the United States, 50-µg Formulations

Brand Name[a]	Estrogen per Tablet (µg)	Total Estrogen (µg)	Progestin Type	Progestin per Tablet (mg)	Total Progestin (mg)	Approximate Norethindrone Equivalents[b] (mg)
Genora 1/50 Norethin 1/50M Norinyl 1+50 Ortho-Novum 1/50	50[c]	1,050	Norethindrone	1.0	21.0	21.0
Ovcon 50	50	1,050	Norethindrone	1.0	21.0	21.0
Norlestrin 1/50	50	1,050	Norethindrone acetate	1.0	21.0	21.0
Norlestrin 2.5/50	50	1,050	Norethindrone acetate	2.5	52.5	52.5
Demulen 1/50	50	1,050	Ethinodiol diacetate	1.0	21.0	21.0
Ovral[d]	50	1,050	Levonorgestrel	0.25	5.25	52.5-105

[a]Regimens of both 21 and 28 days are listed as the same formulation.

[b]Based on estimates of approximate progestin potencies (reviewed by Dorflinger, 1985).

[c]Contains Mestranol, which is metabolized to ethinyl estradiol. Mestranol is generally considered to be equivalent or slightly less potent than ethinyl estradiol.

[d]The total progestin content (norgestrel) is 0.5 mg; however, 50 percent is the inactive enantiomer dextronorgestrel.

TABLE C-3 Summary of Estrogen and Progestin Contents of Phasic Formulations of Oral Contraceptives Available in the United States

Brand Name	Estrogen per Tablet[a] (µg)	Total Estrogen (µg)	Progestin Type	Progestin per Tablet[a] (mg)	Total Progestin (mg)	Approximate Norethindrone Equivalents[b] (mg)
Ortho-Novum 7/7/7	35(21)	735	Norethindrone	0.5(7) 0.75(7) 1.0(7)	15.75	15.75
Tri-Norinyl	35(21)	735	Norethindrone	0.5(7) 1.0(9) 0.5(5)	15.0	15.0
Ortho-Novum 10/11	35(21)	735	Norethindrone	0.5(10) 1.0(11)	16.0	16.0
Tri-Levlen Triphasil	30(6) 40(5) 30(10)	680	Levonorgestrel	0.50(6) 0.075(5) 0.125(10)	1.925	19.25-38.5

[a]Number of days at each dose.

[b]Based on estimates of approximate progestin potencies (Dorflinger, 1985).

chemically related to levonorgestrel and norethindrone. Femodene contains gestodene, the most potent progestin used in oral contraceptives. Marvelon contains the progestin desogestrel, which is transformed into its active form, 3-keto-desogestrel, after ingestion. Cilest contains norgestimate, which is active in its parent form but which is also metabolized to a number of metabolites, including levonorgestrel, that have biological activity. In addition to the monophasic forms, the triphasic forms of each of these oral contraceptives will most likely also become available (see Table C-4).

Publications and promotional materials on each of these new progestins have been extensive for the monophasic formulations (except Cilest), and discuss the similarities and putative advantages over the other currently available formulations. In reality, the clinical profiles, when compared with those of the norethindrone and levonorgestrel triphasics, are quite similar (Chez, 1989). The contraceptive effectiveness of these formulations is high—generally less than one pregnancy per 100 woman-years. Cycle control may be slightly better with the gestodene preparation, and slightly poorer with the desogestrel formulation, than is possible with the currently available triphasics

TABLE C-4 Summary of Estrogen and Progestin Contents of Potential New U.S. Oral Contraceptive Formulations

Brand Name[a]	Estrogen per Tablet[b] (μg)	Total Estrogen (μg)	Progestin Type	Progestin per Tablet[b] (mg)	Total Progestin (mg)
Cilest	35	735	Norgestimate	0.25	5.25
Marvelon	30	630	Desogestrel[c]	0.15	3.15
Femodene	30	630	Gestodene	0.075	1.575
Triphasic Cilest	35	735	Norgestimate	0.180(7) 0.215(7) 0.250(7)	4.515
Triphasic Femodene	30(6) 40(5) 30(10)	680	Gestodene	0.05(6) 0.07(5) 0.10(10)	1.67
Triphasic Marvelon	35(7) 30(7) 30(7)	665	Desogestrel	0.05(7) 0.10(7) 0.15(7)	2.10

[a]Current European brand names, which will not necessarily be used in the United States once the formulations are approved for marketing.

[b]Number of days at each dose.

[c]Desogestrel must be metabolized to 3-keto-desogestrel to be active.

and low-dose monophasics (Chez, 1989). However, good comparative data on these formulations and cycle control are not available, and a definitive statement cannot be made without such comparative studies.

The major metabolic feature that seems to set these formulations apart from older formulations, particularly the desogestrel formulation, appears to be a greater overall estrogenicity. That is, the ability of the progestins in the doses provided to counterbalance many estrogen-regulated actions, mediated by the inherent androgenicity and antiestrogenicity of the progestin, is less. Changes in sex hormone-binding globulin (SHBG) are one indicator of the estrogen/androgen balance of a formulation. SHBG approximately triples with desogestrel and norgestimate formulations, doubles or triples with the gestodene formulation, and increases twofold or less with the triphasic levonorgestrel formulation (Chez, 1989). Finally, extensive research on lipid changes, which also reflect the estrogen/androgen balance, similarly suggests an estrogen-dominant effect of the new formulations.

In both animal and human studies, gestodene has been shown to be the most progestogenic steroid, followed by 3-keto-desogestrel, levonorgestrel, norgestimate, and norethindrone. Many of the unwanted side effects of oral contraceptives relate to the inherent androgenic activity of their components (both through a direct effect and indirectly, by displacing endogenous androgens from SHBG). Consequently, researchers have compared the relative androgenicity of these progestins both in animal studies and receptor-binding assays. The results indicate that, overall, levonorgestrel is the most androgenic and gestodene is similar or slightly less androgenic, followed by 3-keto-desogestrel and norethindrone. Norgestimate has not been directly compared with the other progestins but is essentially devoid of androgenic activity.

Kloosterboer and colleagues (1988) have calculated what they term a selectivity index, defined as the ratio of the relative binding affinity of each progestin for the progesterone receptor and the relative binding affinity for the androgen receptor. These authors reported that the selectivity index for 3-keto-desogestrel is the highest, followed by gestodene, levonorgestrel, and norethindrone; the study did not report on norgestimate. When compared with levonorgestrel, gestodene is about three times more selective for the progesterone receptor (i.e., at the same dose, given similar bioavailability, gestodene should have about one-third the relative androgenic effect). The selectivity ratio for 3-keto-desogestrel is three to five that of levonorgestrel. Thus, for example, because the dose of estrogen and progestin in Marvelon and Nordette are the same, one might predict the 3-keto-desogestrel formulation (Marvelon) would be markedly less androgenic. This speculation is confirmed in the literature in studies that examine changes in lipids or SHBG.

In a direct comparison of Marvelon and Femodene, there were no differences in 19 parameters of lipid metabolism, gonadotropins, pro-lactin, ovarian and adrenal steroids, and SHBG (Jung-Hoffmann et al., 1988). Like Femodene and Marvelon, the Cilest formulation appears to have little impact on the overall lipid profile, and any reported changes are in a positive direction (e.g., high-density lipoprotein [HDL]-cholesterol increases slightly and there is an improved HDL/low-density lipoprotein [LDL] ratio).

An oral contraceptive containing progestogen and melatonin is presently undergoing phase 1 and 2 clinical trials (with phase 3 trials scheduled to begin in early 1991) in the Netherlands. If contraceptive effectiveness can be demonstrated, large-scale use may provide appropriate observational data to test the hypothesis (Cohen et al., 1978) that melatonin protects against breast cancer in perimenopausal women. The combination of hypothalamic-releasing agents with low doses of progestogen has also been suggested as a possible contraceptive modality that would reduce the incidence not only of ovarian and uterine cancer but of breast cancer (Pike et al., 1989). There is insufficient clinical experience to confirm or refute these hypotheses.

IMPLICATIONS FOR RESEARCH

Most of the epidemiological studies to date have provided information exclusively on long-term use of older oral contraceptive formulations that had high total steroid doses. Limited information is available on long-term use of lower-dose formulations, particularly as related to breast cancer, and nothing is known about the triphasic formulations. The new progestin formulations will further complicate the study of the relationship of long-term use of the pill from an early age and breast cancer.

Three important considerations with respect to studies of the potential link of oral contraceptives (and specific oral contraceptive formulations) and breast cancer loom large for the 1990s. First, there is wide variation among individuals in blood levels of ethinyl estradiol and the progestin component of an oral contractive following oral administration (Goebelsmann, 1986; Kuhl et al., 1988, Jung-Hoffman et al., 1988; Goldzieher, 1990). Given this individual variation in absorption and metabolism for each component, the average estrogen/progestin ratio will vary for each individual and may be different than that calculated from the oral contraceptive steroid dose. As a result, the composite effect at the level of the breast may vary among individuals, and within an individual over time. A question is whether this individual variation in estrogen-to-progestin ratio over months or years may in some way alter the predisposition of various women to develop breast cancer—if, in fact, the putative association of long-term early use and increased relative risk holds up. The answer to this question rests in a better understanding of the interaction of estrogen and progestin in normal breast tissue. In addition, although new biological indicators are being studied in an attempt to unravel the etiology of breast cancer, and the potential linkage of oral contraceptive use with breast cancer, pharmacokinetic and pharmacodynamic differences in the way individual women handle steroids should not be overlooked and merit further research.

Second, one of the features suggested as a major advantage of the new progestins is that their total steroid content is generally lower than that of many currently available formulations. Pharmacologically and physiologically, however, this benefit may be a red herring because these new progestins are more potent than current formulations in eliciting their effects. Therefore, a lower dose produces the same antiovulatory effect, as well as the same effect on a number of other progestin-regulated parameters. There may be some differential effects of these progestins at the level of the uterus, however, in addition to a distinction in their inherent androgenicity or antiestrogenicity. Androgens have been found to inhibit estrogen-stimulated growth and reverse estrogen inhibition of a progesterone-binding breast cyst protein (GCDFP-24) by human breast cancer cells (Simard et al., 1990). If this effect holds for normal mammary tissue, the inherent androgenicity or antiestrogenicity of the progestin in oral contraceptive formulations might play a role in balancing estrogen-stimulated growth effects. This issue merits closer scrutiny and additional research.

How the progestogenic activity of each progestin enters this equation is unknown. Progestins are known to antagonize estrogen action, at least in part, through down-regulation of the estrogen receptor. A recent study using breast cancer cells in culture (Alexander et al., 1990) demonstrated that this down-regulation was linked to inhibition of estrogen action. A number of questions follow from this research. Is this effect the same in normal breast tissue as in breast cancer cells? Is the effect the same in various cell types of the breast (see Chapter 3)? Does ethinyl estradiol have the same effect as estradiol at the receptor level? How does receptor regulation differ with continuous and simultaneous administration of estrogen and progestin, as opposed to the normal cycle? What is the effect of changing the ratio of estrogen and progestin (i.e., different pill types, different absorption and metabolism)? The interrelationship of estrogen, progestins, and androgens, particularly in normal breast tissue, is a priority area of research.

Third, the currently available triphasics, as well as the new progestin formulations, have now become more estrogen dominant than many (although not all) of the low-estrogen oral contraceptives. One recent report indicates that increased estrogen content of oral contraceptive formulations is positively associated with an increased thymidine labeling index, an indicator of cell proliferation (Anderson et al., 1989). In that study, information was most complete for levonorgestrel- and norethindrone-containing formulations. A key question is whether it is the total estrogen content or the estrogen dominance of a formulation that is most important as far as this indicator is concerned. If possible, the effects of new formulations on thymidine labeling index rates should be studied carefully and compared with triphasics and other currently available low-estrogen oral contraceptives.

In summary, four questions related to oral contraceptive formulation stand as top research priorities for the 1990s. Do individual variations in blood levels in ethinyl estradiol and the progestin component of oral contraceptives affect risk of breast cancer? What are the effects of the progestin component of the pill in modulating estrogen action? Do the inherent androgenic or antiestrogenic properties of different oral contraceptive formulations affect normal breast tissue response? How will the overall estrogen dominance of the new oral contraceptives affect breast tissue response?

REFERENCES

Alexander, I. E., J. Shine, and R. L. Sutherland. 1990. Progestin regulation of estrogen receptor messenger RNA in human breast cancer cells. Molecular Endocrinology 4:821-828.

Anderson, T. J., S. Battersby, R. J. B. King, K. McPherson, and J. J. Going. 1989. Oral contraceptive use influences resting breast proliferation. Human Pathology 20:1139-1144.

Chez, R. A. 1989. Clinical aspects of three new progestogens: Desogestrel, gestodene, and norgestimate. American Journal of Obstetrics and Gynecology 160:1292-1300.

Cohen, M., M. Lippman, and B. Chabner. 1978. Role of pineal gland in aetiology and treatment of breast cancer. Lancet 2:814-816.

Contraceptive Technology Update. 1989. Triphasics trendy—but what are actual benefits? Vol. 10, pp. 161-173.

Dorflinger, L. J. 1985. Relative potency of progestins used in oral contraceptives. Contraception 31:557-570.

Goebelsmann, U. 1986. Pharmacokinetics of contraceptive steroids in humans. Pp. 67-111 in Contraceptive Steroids: Pharmacology and Safety, A. T. Gregoire and R. T. Blye, eds. New York: Plenum Press.

Goldzieher, J. W. 1990. Selected aspects of the pharmacokinetics and metabolism of ethinyl estrogens and their clinical application. American Journal of Obstetrics and Gynecology 163:318-322.

Jung-Hoffmann, C., F. Heidt, and H. Kuhl. 1988. Effect of two oral contraceptives containing 30 µg ethinylestradiol and 75 µg gestodene or 150 µg desogestrel upon various hormonal parameters. Contraception 38:593-603.

Kloosterboer, H. J., C. A. Vonk-Noordegraaf, and E. W. Turpijn. 1988. Selectivity in progesterone and androgen receptor binding of progestagens used in oral contraceptives. Contraception 38:325-332.

Kuhl, H., C. Jung-Hoffmann, and F. Heidt. 1988a. Serum levels of 3-keto-desogestrel and SHBG during 12 cycles of treatment with 30 µg ethinylestradiol and 150 µg desogestrel. Contraception 38:381-390.

Kuhl, H., C. Jung-Hoffmann, and F. Heidt. 1988b. Alterations in the serum levels of gestodene and SHBG during 12 cycles of treatment with 30 µg ethinylestradiol and 75 µg gestodene. Contraception 38:477-486.

Pike, M. C., R. K. Ross, R. A. Lobo, T. J. A. Key, M. Potts, and B. E. Henderson. 1989. LHRH agonists and the prevention of breast and ovarian cancer. British Journal of Cancer 60:142-148.

Simard, J., S. Dauvois, D. E. Haagensen, C. Levesque, Y. Merand, and F. Labrie. 1990. Regulation of progesterone-binding breast cyst protein GCDFP-24 secretion by estrogens and androgens in human breast cancer cells: A new marker of steroid action in breast cancer. Endocrinology 126:3223-3231.

D
Animal Models of Sex Steroid Hormones and Mammary Cancer: Lessons for Understanding Studies in Humans

DIANA B. PETITTI

For many years, studies in animals have been used to evaluate the carcinogenicity of various chemicals, including drugs. The effect of chemicals on the occurrence of cancer in animals is the basis for regulating human exposure in the workplace, in the environment, in food, and in pharmaceuticals. Studies of cancer in animals are often the sole input to the growing field of risk assessment. Most important, animal models of cancer have provided useful insights into the mechanisms of chemical carcinogenesis that have enlarged our understanding of the biology of human cancer.

The effect of various sex steroid hormones on the occurrence of mammary cancer has been studied in a variety of species, but the most extensive studies have been conducted in mice, rats, and beagle dogs. There have also been some studies in monkeys, which were conducted on a scale considered large for such studies. The low spontaneous rate of mammary tumors in primates, however, seriously limits the usefulness of the monkey as a model for studying sex steroid hormones and mammary cancer.

In theory, sex steroid hormones might cause mammary cancer because they are intrinsically carcinogenic or because they have hormonal effects that lead to cancer (Roe, 1976). This paper considers studies in mice, rats, and beagle dogs that were designed as direct

Diana B. Petitti is an associate professor in the Department of Family and Community Medicine, in the School of Medicine, University of California, San Francisco.

tests of the carcinogenicity of sex steroid hormones. It also reviews studies in these three species designed to elucidate the hormonal mechanisms of mammary cancer in general and in relation to exogenous administration of sex steroid hormones.

DIRECT TESTS OF CARCINOGENICITY

When the first steroid contraceptives were developed, they were submitted to the same toxicological tests that had been routinely conducted with other drugs. These tests were performed to identify the acute and chronic toxic effects of the drugs, and they were generally carried out in one rodent and one nonrodent species.

Because contraceptive steroids were to be taken by a large number of healthy young women for a considerable length of time, and because many important cancers in women were considered to be hormonally mediated, the carcinogenic risk of contraceptive steroids was of particular concern. This concern led the U.S. Food and Drug Administration (FDA) to require long-term tests of tumorigenicity in at least two species as a precondition for marketing approval. Later, FDA and other drug regulatory agencies began to require additional evaluation of contraceptive steroids in long-term studies in beagle dogs and rhesus monkeys.

Information from the long-term tests conducted to obtain marketing approval constitutes a valuable data resource and is reviewed here in some depth. It is important to recognize, however, that in 1932, Lacassagne (1932) demonstrated that exogenous estrogens caused mammary cancer in mice. By the late 1950s, it was already well established that exogenous estrogens caused mammary cancer in at least some strains of mice and rats.

Mice and Rats

A 1972 report by the U.K. Committee on Safety of Medicines (CSM, 1972) constitutes the largest data base on tumorigenicity of contraceptive steroids in mice and rats. The studies reported by the CSM involved 7,000 mice and 6,500 rats who were given six different estrogen/progestogen combinations at three doses and were examined for the presence or absence of neoplasia at 18 different sites. The tests of different estrogens and estrogen/progestogen combinations were carried out according to a standard protocol. Almost all experiments in mice used the CF-LP mouse strain; all of the experiments used 120 mice per treatment group. Doses of contraceptive steroids were 2-5, 50, and 200-400 times the human contraceptive dose. The rat experiments used the same three dose groups, but the strain of rat and the number of rats per dose group varied from experiment to experiment.

The CSM report itself presented no tests of statistical significance in the comparisons of tumors in the treated and control animals. The analysis presented in the CSM report also did not take into account mortality during the course of the experiment, nor was any attempt made to determine whether there were dose-response relationships. These problems hamper interpretations of the results of the study, but the information is useful depite its limitations.

Mice who were treated with estrogen alone showed no excess of malignant mammary tumors. Mice treated with any of the six progestogens alone or with any of the combinations of estrogen and progestogen also showed no excess of malignant mammary tumors. In some experiements, female rats treated with ethinyl estradiol or mestranol alone had an increase in malignant mammary tumors (Table D-1). An excess of malignant mammary tumors also appeared in male rats treated with norethynodrel alone (Table D-2). In both male and female rats, an increase in malignant mammary tumors occurred following treatment with a norethynodrel/mestranol combination and norethindrone/mestranol combination, but not following treatment with other combinations (Table D-3). Female rats showed an excess of malignant mammary tumors following treatment with a combination of ethynodiol diacetate and mestranol.

Review of these experiments leads to several conclusions. First, estrogens alone, some progestogens, and some estrogen/progestogen combinations cause an increase in the occurrence of malignant mammary tumors in at least some strains of rats and mice. Second, there is strong evidence that progestogens modify the effect of estrogen on the occurrence of malignant mammary tumors in rats, as is also shown in experiments by other investigators (Schardein, 1980). Last, the effects of estrogens and progestogens on mammary cancer in mice and rats are strain specific (see also Rudali et al., 1971).

Beagle Dogs

The FDA began to require long-term studies of contraceptive steroids in beagles as a precondition for approval for marketing following the observation that one progestogen (MK-665, or ethynerone) caused high rates of mammary tumors in beagles even at doses that were a low multiple of the human contraceptive dose. Benign mammary tumors are considered an established precursor of malignant mammary tumors in beagles, and the beagle mammary response to

TABLE D-1   Malignant Mammary Tumors in Rats Treated with Mestranol or Ethinyl Estradiol Alone

Experiment	Percent Increase	
	Males	Females
8	N.a.	16.7
8	N.a.	19.2
10	N.a.	0.9
11	0.0	2.6
12	1.4	3.7

N.a.: Not applicable.
SOURCE: Committee on Safety of Medicines, 1972.

TABLE D-2   Malignant Mammary Tumors in Rats Treated with Various Progestogens Alone

Progestogen	Percent Increase	
	Males	Females
Norethynodrel	15.0	2.5
Norethindrone	4.2	2.5
Chlormadinone acetate	0.0	2.7
Lynestrenol	N.a.	2.6
dl Norgestrel	0.0	0.0
Megestrol acetate	0.0	4.1

N.a.: Not applicable.
SOURCE: Committee on Safety of Medicines, 1972.

TABLE D-3   Malignant Mammary Tumors in Rats Treated with Estrogen/Progestogen Combinations

Combination[a]	Percent Increase	
	Males	Females
Norethynodrel + Mestranol	19.2	14.3
Ethyno/idiol diacetate + Mestranol	4.2	15.0
Norethindrone acetate + Ethinyl estradiol	0.0	2.1
Norethindrone + Mestranol	11.7	25.5
dl Norgestrel + Ethinyl estradiol	0.0	0.7
Megestrol acetate + Ethinyl estradiol	4.1	6.3

[a]High-dose levels.
SOURCE: Committee on Safety of Medicines, 1972.

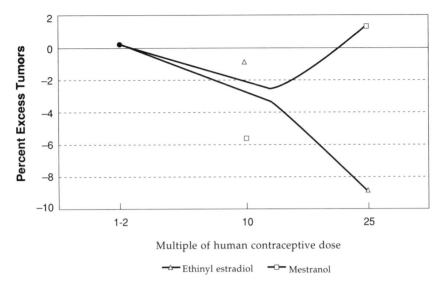

FIGURE D-1   Excess percentage of dogs with tumors. SOURCE: Larsson and Machin (1989).

progestogen was considered a promising screening test for mammary carcinogenicity of contraceptive steroids.

Much has been written about the appropriateness, and inappropriateness, of the beagle as a model for studying the carcinogenicity of steroid hormones in humans (see El Etreby et al., 1979, 1989). These arguments are discussed later. First, however, let us consider the findings of studies in beagles that were summarized in a systematic form by Larsson and Machin (1989) for a conference sponsored by the World Health Organization (held in Geneva, Switzerland in January 1987). These studies are representative of the other published studies of sex steroid hormones and mammary tumors in beagles.

The experimental studies were all carried out according to a standard protocol. Three dose groups of 1-2, 10, and 25 times the human contraceptive dose were used in each experiment, together with an untreated control group. The mandated minimum number of dogs in each dose group and in the control group was 12; most experiments included 16 or 20 dogs in each group. All dogs were treated and followed for seven years, half the estimated life span of the beagle. Because even relatively low doses of some progestogens cause fatal pyometria in beagles, all experimental animals were hysterectomized.

Larsson and Machin (1989) compiled the results of 26 different

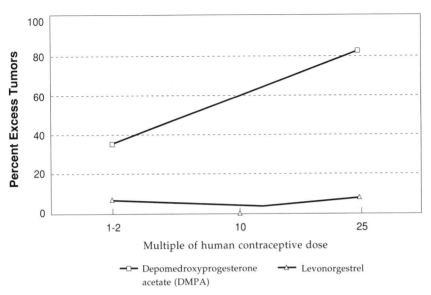

FIGURE D-2 Excess percentage of dogs with tumors. SOURCE: Larsson and Machin (1989).

experiments using estrogen, various progestogens, and estrogen/progestogen combinations. These experiments involved mestranol and ethinyl estradiol given alone and 16 different progestogens, both alone and in combination with mestranol or ethinyl estradiol. In the beagle, neither ethinyl estradiol nor mestranol alone caused an increase in mammary tumors, as shown in Figure D-1, which gives the excess percentage of dogs with tumors following treatment with ethinyl estradiol and mestranol for three multiples of the human contraceptive dose. Statistical analysis of these data taking into account survival time and dose-response yields the same conclusion about the mammary tumorigenicity of estrogen alone in beagle dogs (Larsson and Machin, 1989).

The beagle dog as a model for studying the mammary carcinogenicity of contraceptive steroids came under close scrutiny because of observations of the effects of depomedroxyprogesterone acetate (DMPA) in this system. The profound tumorigenic effect of DMPA in beagles is illustrated in Figure D-2, which again gives the excess percentage of dogs with tumors following treatment with DMPA at several multiples of the human contraceptive dose. The figure and analysis show that DMPA is a potent mammary tumorigen at doses that are close to the human contraceptive dose, whereas levonorgestrel shows almost

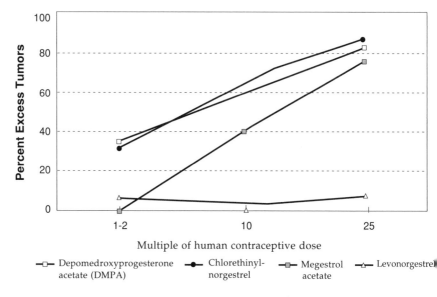

FIGURE D-3 Excess percentage of dogs with tumors. SOURCE: Larsson and Machin (1989).

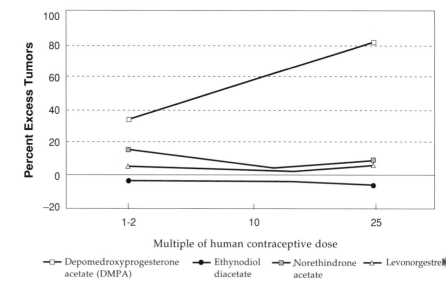

FIGURE D-4 Excess percentage of dogs with tumors. SOURCE: Larsson and Machin (1989).

no effect on mammary tumorigenesis in the beagle in doses that are the same multiple of the human contraceptive dose. Again, statistical techniques that take into account survival of the dogs and dose-response yield the same conclusion (Larsson and Machin, 1989).

Figures D-3 and D-4 illustrate further the variability in mammary tumorigenicity of different progestogens in beagles. Leaving DMPA and levonorgestrel as "reference" compounds, Figure D-3 shows the excess percentage of tumors after treatment with two C-21 hydroxy progestogens—chlorethinyl norgestrel and megestrol. Both are potent mammary tumorigens in beagles. In contrast, Figure D-4 shows that, like levonorgestrel, norethindrone acetate and ethynodiol diacetate do not cause an excess of mammary tumors in beagles even at high multiples of the human contraceptive dose. It is noteworthy that progesterone and medroxyprogesterone acetate are, like DMPA, potent mammary tumorigens in the beagle (Figure D-5).

Overall, the data support the conclusion that there are important differences in the mammary tumorigenicity of different progestogens in the beagle at comparable multiples of the human contraceptive dose.

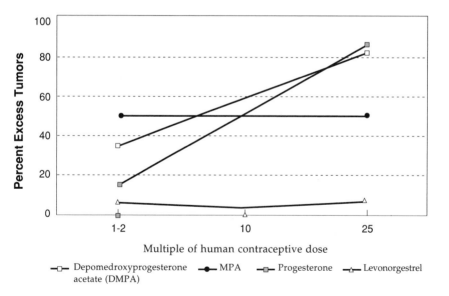

FIGURE D-5 Excess percentage of dogs with tumors. SOURCE: Larsson and Machin (1989).

PHARMACOKINETICS OF VARIOUS STEROIDS
IN MICE, RATS, AND BEAGLES

Many of the arguments against use of the beagle as a model for studying the carcinogenicity of progestogens in humans center on a consideration of differences between dogs and humans in the pharmacokinetics of the steroids. A careful, direct comparative study of the pharmacokinetics of five steroids in rats, beagles, and humans was reported by Humpel (1989), who confirmed that there were both important similarities and important differences in various pharmacokinetic parameters between dogs and humans. This study also showed, however, that the pharmacokinetics of the five steroids were different in rats and humans. Thus, a consideration of differences between humans and other species in the pharmacokinetics of various steroids would lead one to reject the rat as well as the dog as a model for studying these compounds. For this reason, data from the experiments reported by the U. K.'s Committee on Safety of Medicines are no more reassuring about the effects of steroid hormones and mammary cancer than the beagle experiments are alarming.

An elegant experiment in beagles done by El Etreby and colleagues (1989) gives considerable insight into the mechanism for differences in mammary tumorigenicity of the various progestogens in the beagle. In this important experiment, the investigators explored the relationship between progestogen dose and mammary tumor response using doses of several progestogens that were larger or smaller than the "standard" multiples of the human contraceptive dose. They were able to show that all of the progestogens tested were mammary tumorigens. The difference in mammary tumorigenicity of various progestogens was a matter of the dose at which the effect occurred and not a matter of some progestogens causing mammary tumors and some not causing mammary tumors. Levonorgestrel, which is very poorly absorbed by the dog, showed high rates of mammary tumorigenicity but only at doses that are many hundreds of times a multiple of the human contraceptive dose.

STUDIES OF MECHANISMS FOR MAMMARY
CARCINOGENICITY OF SEX STEROID HORMONES
IN MICE, RATS, AND DOGS

The most important lessons from animal studies of sex steroids come not from what must be considered fairly crude attempts to study their intrinsic carcinogenicity, but from studies that have gone further to define the mechanisms for steroid-induced mammary car-

TABLE D-4 Effect of Median Eminence Lesions on Prolactin Levels and Mammary Tumors in Rats

	Effect	
Treatment	Prolactin	Percent Tumors
Control	50.9	19.0
Median eminence	179.8	52.2

SOURCE: Welsch et al., 1970.

cinogenicity in mice, rats, and beagles. It is now agreed that estrogen-induced mammary tumors in rats and mice are caused by increased levels of prolactin, which are a consequence of estrogen-induced benign pituitary adenomas. Thus, Welsch (1970) showed that lesions in the hypothalamus of the rat that destroyed inhibitors of pituitary prolactin release led both to increases in levels of prolactin and increases in malignant mammary tumors (Table D-4). Subsequently, Welsch (1977) showed that estrogen-induced mammary tumors in mice are prevented by simultaneous administration of a prolactin inhibitor, 2-bromo-α-ergocryptine (Table D-5). This prolactin inhibitor also prevented mammary tumors caused by simultaneous administration of estrogen and progestogen (Table D-6).

Studies in beagles have implicated progestogen-induced elevations in growth hormone in the pathogenesis of mammary tumors seen in experiments in dogs. Similar to the studies in rats and mice, this link rests first on the demonstration that progestogens that cause mammary tumors elevate growth hormone levels (Table D-7; Concannon et al., 1980). Later, El Etreby and coworkers (1989) showed that inhi-

TABLE D-5 Mammary Tumors in Mice After Treatment with Estrogen Alone and Estrogen Plus Prolactin Inhibitor[a]

Treatment	Percentage with Tumors
Control	11.0
Ethinyl estradiol	27.3
Ethinyl estradiol + CB-154[a]	9.0

[a]CB-154 = 12-bromo-α-ergocryptine.
SOURCE: Welsch et al., 1977.

TABLE D-6 Mammary Tumors in Mice After Treatment with Enovid Mestranol (plus Norethynodrel) Alone and Enovid Plus[a] Prolactin Inhibitor

Treatment	Percentage with Tumors
Control	14.0
Enovid	30.0
Enovid + CB-154[a]	10.0

[a]CB-154 = 2-bromo-α-ergocryptine.
SOURCE: Welsch et al., 1977.

TABLE D-7 Serum Hormone Levels in Beagles After Treatment with Progesterone and Medroxyprogesterone Acetate (MPA)

Hormone	Control	Progesterone[a]	MPA[b]
Cortisol	13.7	14.9	1.7
Prolactin	12.6	13.6	13.7
Growth hormone	0.4	0.6	9.5

[a]"Physiologic dose."
[b]Dose = milligrams per kilogram for 3 months.
SOURCE: Concannon et al., 1980.

bition of progestogen-induced increases of growth hormone altered the beagle mammary response to the progestogen (data not shown).

CONCLUSIONS

Studies of the relationship of sex steriod hormones and mammary cancer in mice, rats, and beagles point to three main conclusions that apply to all three species. 1. Either estrogen alone, progestogen alone, or a combination of estrogen and progestogen have been shown to be mammary carcinogens. 2. The effect of estrogen on mammary cancer can be modified by the progestogen. 3. The mammary carcinogenic effects of sex steroid hormones are mediated by an effect of the sex steroid on a pituitary hormone, which is the mammary mitogen. This last observation, the most important, draws attention to a hypothesis put forth by El Etreby and colleagues (1989) that progestogen and

TABLE D-8 Comparison of Risk Factors for Mammary Cancer in Mice, Rats, Dogs, and Humans

Risk Factor	Mice	Rats	Dogs	Humans
Increasing age	↑	↑	↑	↑
Higher age at first pregnancy	?	?	?	↑
Ever pregnant	?	?	↓	↓
Oophorectomy	?	?	↓	↓
Obesity	↑	↑	↑	↑

? = not studied; ↑ = increased; ↓ = decreased.

estrogen in humans might affect mammary tumors through their effect on a novel pituitary mammary mitogen.

INTERESTING QUESTIONS RAISED BY ANIMAL STUDIES

A comparison of information about mammary cancer in mice, rats, beagles, and humans (Table D-8) shows that our knowledge of risk factors for mammary cancer in mice and rats is very poor. It would be easier to judge how much one could extrapolate between these two species and humans if there was as much information about spontaneous mammary cancer in these animals as there was for humans.

Consideration of both the epidemiology of mammary cancer in animals, including humans, and the material presented here raises some interesting questions. Does pregnancy alter the risk of mammary cancer in rats and mice? If so, does it do so by altering prolactin levels, suggesting that prolactin is a unifying mechanism for mammary cancer in mice and rats? Similarly, are increasing rates of mammary cancer with age in free-living beagle dogs accompanied by increasing levels of growth hormone? Are endogenous levels of prolactin predictive of mammary cancer in rats and mice, and are endogenous levels of growth hormone predictive of mammary cancer in beagles? Do estrogens, progestogens, and estrogen/progestogen combinations affect prolactin levels and growth hormone levels in humans? Last, if progestogens importantly modify the effect of estrogen on mammary carcinogenesis of sex steroid in mice, rats, and dogs, is it possible that the secular changes in the balance of estrogen and progestogen in commonly used oral contraceptives in different places explain differences in some of the risk estimates that have been derived from these studies?

Better integration of information from animal studies of mammary cancer and steroid contraceptives with thinking about human epidemiological data would undoubtedly advance our understanding of the epidemiological data. Similarly, epidemiological approaches to the study of mammary cancer in animals would help establish the suitability and unsuitability of the animal models for humans.

REFERENCES

Committee on Safety of Medicines (CSM). 1972. Carcinogenicity Tests of Oral Contraceptives. London: Her Majesty's Stationery Office.

Concannon, P., N. Altszuler, J. Hampshire, W. R. Butler, and W. Hansel. 1980. Growth hormone, prolactin, and cortisol in dogs developing mammary nodules and an acromegaly-like appearance during treatment with medroxyprogesterone acetate. Endocrinology 106:1173-1177.

El Etreby, M. F., K.-J. Graf, S. Beier, W. Elger, P. Gunzel, and F. Neumann. 1979. Suitability of the beagle dog as a test model for the tumorigenic potential of contraceptive steroids: A short review. Contraception 20:237-256.

El Etreby, M. F., S. Beier, and P. Gunzel. 1989. Comparative endocrine pharmacodynamics of contraceptive steroids. Pp. 179-192 in Safety Requirements for Contraceptive Steroids, F. Michal, ed. Cambridge: Cambridge University Press.

Humpel, M. 1989. Comparative pharmacokinetics of selected steroids in animal species and man. Pp. 193-210 in Safety Requirements for Contraceptive Steroids, F. Michal, ed. Cambridge: Cambridge University Press.

Lacassagne, A. L. 1932. Apparition de cancers de la mamelle chez la souris malé soumise à des injections de folliculine. Comptes Rendus des Séances de la Société de Biologie et des Filiales 195:632-638.

Larsson, K. S., and D. Machin. 1989. Predictability of the safety of hormonal contraceptives from canine toxicological studies. Pp. 230-269 in Safety Requirements for Contraceptive Steroids, F. Michal, ed. Cambridge: Cambridge University Press.

Roe, F. 1976. Possible carcinogenic hazards of oral contraception. Proceedings of the Royal Society of Medicine 69:349-350.

Rudali, G., E. Coezy, F. Frederic, and F. Apiou. 1971. Susceptibility of mice of different strains to the mammary carcinogenic action of natural and synthetic oestrogens. Revue Europeene d'Estudes Cliniques et Biologiques 16:425-439.

Schardein, J. L. 1980. Studies of the components of an oral contraceptive in albino rats. 2. Progestogenic component and comparison of effects of the components and the combined agent. Journal of Toxicology and Environmental Health 6:895-906.

Welsch, C. W., H. Hagasawa, and J. Meites. 1970. Increased incidence of spontaneous mammary tumors in female rats with induced hypothalamic lesions. Cancer Research 30:2310-2313.

Welsch, C. W., C. Adams, L. K. Lambrecht, C. C. Hassett, and C. L. Brooks. 1977. 17-β-oestradiol and enovid mammary tumorigenesis in c3H/HeJ female mice: Counteraction by concurrent 2-bromo-α-ergocryptine. British Journal of Cancer 35:322-328.

E

Risks and Benefits of Oral Contraceptives: Will Breast Cancer Tip the Balance?

DAVID C. G. SKEGG

Concern about breast cancer is the main cloud hanging over oral contraceptives. When they were first marketed three decades ago, some hoped they might reduce the risk of breast cancer. The Puerto Rico contraceptive study, instigated by Gregory Pincus in 1961, was intended to explore the "anticancer effect on the breast and genital system" of using the pill (Potts et al., 1982). The recognition that oral contraceptives reduced the risk of benign breast disease fueled the hope that they would also protect against breast cancer. The great majority of studies, however, have shown no alteration of risk; indeed, several recent investigations have suggested that oral contraceptives may increase the risk of breast cancer in certain groups of women (Schlesselman, 1989; Thomas, 1989; Mann, 1990). The current decline in oral contraceptive use by American women has been attributed to media publicity about these positive studies (Contraception Report, 1990).

Because breast cancer is so common, with a cumulative incidence rate (before age 75) of about 9 percent in the United States (Muir et al., 1987), any general increase in risk associated with a widely used method of contraception would be of serious concern. Breast cancer also happens to be a disease that women and their families particu-

David C. G. Skegg, University of Otago Medical School, Dunedin, New Zealand.

larly fear, so any increase in risk might carry a disproportionate weight when choices about contraception are being made. Nevertheless, women and their physicians need to weigh up all of the benefits and risks of oral contraceptives, and to decide whether any increased risk of breast cancer is likely to tip the balance. To do this, it is necessary to consider the range of breast cancer effects that might plausibly emerge over the next few decades.

ESTABLISHED BENEFITS AND RISKS

The outstanding benefit of oral contraception is its prevention of unplanned pregnancy—with such a high degree of effectiveness, convenience, and reversibility (Ory et al., 1983). Future historians will attempt to assess the pill's enormous range of influences on twentieth-century society. From a medical point of view, the effectiveness of the pill is of greatest significance to women in developing countries. Whereas maternal mortality is something many of us read about in Victorian novels, it is still a grim reality in developing countries. Each year pregnancy and childbirth claim the lives of at least half a million women (Royston and Armstrong, 1989). A new World Health Organization report estimates that, in Bali, a woman has a 1-in-32 lifetime risk of dying from pregnancy-related causes; in Bangladesh the risk is 1-in-26, and in parts of rural Africa (where high maternal mortality rates coexist with high fertility) it may be as high as 1 in 15 (Royston and Armstrong, 1989). By preventing unwanted pregnancies and enabling women to space births, the pill contributes not only to maternal health but also to the survival and health of children.

Apart from the prevention of pregnancy, oral contraceptives have a wide range of benefits and risks. The noncontraceptive benefits of combined oral contraceptives include reductions in the incidence of menstrual problems (such as dysmenorrhea and menorrhagia), iron-deficiency anemia, pelvic inflammatory disease, functional ovarian cysts, benign breast disease, epithelial ovarian cancer, and endometrial cancer (Prentice and Thomas, 1987; Population Information Program, 1988; Vessey, 1990). The pill's strong protective effects against cancers of the ovary and endometrium are especially important because the protection appears to persist in ex-users for at least 15 years after stopping oral contraception (Cancer and Steroid Hormone Study, 1987a,b).

The most important adverse effects of combined oral contraceptives are their propensity to cause cardiovascular events such as myocardial infarction, thrombotic stroke, hemorrhagic stroke, and venous thrombosis and embolism (Stadel, 1981; Prentice and Thomas, 1987).

Fortunately, these complications are rare and largely confined to current users of oral contraceptives. The increased risk of myocardial infarction is found mainly in women with other risk factors, such as cigarette smoking. The demonstration of these other factors in epidemiological studies has led to much more careful screening of candidates for oral contraception, with the result that many of these catastrophic occurrences are now avoided. It should also be noted that our estimates of cardiovascular risks are based on studies that were carried out in the 1970s, and it is suspected (although not yet proven) that modern low-dose oral contraceptives carry lower risks.

Long-term use of the pill increases the risk of hepatocellular adenoma (Rooks et al., 1979) and (probably) hepatocellular carcinoma (Forman et al., 1986; Neuberger et al., 1986), but these conditions are rare in women of childbearing age in the United States. More worrying is an association between long-term use of oral contraceptives and invasive cancer of the cervix (Prentice and Thomas, 1987; Hulka, 1989; Schlesselman, 1989). It is still unclear whether this association reflects a causal relationship or incomplete adjustment for the confounding influences of the sexual behavior of women and their male partners (Swan and Petitti, 1982).

There are many other suspected beneficial and adverse effects of oral contraception that require further research (Prentice and Thomas, 1987; Population Information Program, 1988; Vessey, 1990). The suggestion that use of the pill might increase the risk of contracting human immunodeficiency virus (HIV) infection, based on a study of prostitutes in Nairobi (Simonsen et al., 1990), has not been confirmed.

BALANCE OF BENEFITS AND RISKS

Any comparison of the risks and benefits of oral contraceptives needs to be specific to particular countries or groups of countries, because the balance sheet will be affected by both the underlying incidence of diseases and the risk of maternal mortality. In those developing nations where maternal mortality is high, the effectiveness of the pill in preventing pregnancy will be of overwhelming importance. Even when attention is focused on a single country, the balance of benefits and risks will be different for different groups of women. Thus, the balance will be different for younger and older women, for smokers and nonsmokers, and so on.

Despite such complexities, several authors have tried to draw up balance sheets of benefits and risks (Tietze et al., 1976; Ory et al., 1983; Prentice and Thomas, 1987; Vessey, 1990). Their approaches have inevitable limitations. First, no value is placed on avoidance of the grief of unwanted pregnancy. Pregnancy is counted only as a possible cause of morbidity and death. Second, attention is generally focused on mortality: how could one compare the alleviation of dysmenorrhea in 1,000 women with the causation of a stroke in one woman? On the other hand, counting mortality enables direct comparisons to be made, and the approach can perhaps be defended on the grounds that "death is unequivocal and of overriding importance to the individual" (Doll, 1973).

Vessey recently described a simplified model of mortality that compares users of oral contraceptives and of condoms in the United Kingdom (Vessey, 1990). He assumes that a cohort of one million women start to use combined oral contraceptives at age 16 and that another cohort of one million women decide to rely on the condom from the same age. Both groups of women continue with their chosen method of birth control until the age of 35, when they (or their partners) are sterilized. Follow-up continues to the age of 50. If it is assumed that oral contraceptives do not affect the risk of breast or cervical cancer, the women in the pill cohort do appreciably better, with 1,134 fewer deaths overall (1,240 fewer if lower cardiovascular risks are assumed). The most striking effect is the prevention of 1,400 deaths from ovarian cancer in the oral contraceptive cohort.

If it is assumed that the association between the pill and cervical cancer is causal and that it persists in ex-users, Vessey estimates that the mortality advantage in the oral contraceptive cohort will be reduced by 764 additional deaths from cervical cancer. He then incorporates the positive findings of the recent U.K. National Case-Control Study of oral contraceptives and breast cancer (U.K. National Case-Control Study Group, 1989). If users of the pill have an increased risk of breast cancer up to the age of 35 but not at older ages, he estimates that their mortality advantage will be reduced by 311 additional deaths from breast cancer. But if it is assumed, as some have suggested, that the increased risk of breast cancer observed in the U.K. National Study will persist beyond age 35, the picture looks very different. Assuming that a relative risk of 1.75 in long-term users persists until age 50, the additional number of deaths from breast cancer in the oral contraceptive cohort will not be 311 but 4,157. Hence, a persisting risk of breast cancer would certainly tip the balance against oral contraceptives.

ORAL CONTRACEPTIVES AND BREAST CANCER

How likely or unlikely is this pessimistic scenario? It must be regarded as very unlikely on the evidence to date because, as noted in other reviews (Schlesselman et al., 1989; Thomas, 1989), the results of case-control and cohort studies in middle-aged women have been reassuringly negative. Some commentators, however, have suggested that a new phenomenon may be emerging (McPherson et al., 1986; Lund, 1989).

Interpreting the positive findings in several recent case-control studies is difficult for two main reasons. The first problem is one of shifting goalposts: the positive subgroups keep changing. For example, Pike's group in Los Angeles reported in 1981 that women who used the pill before their first full-term pregnancy had an increased risk of breast cancer at a young age (Pike et al., 1981). Oral contraceptive use after the first pregnancy was not associated with any change in risk. In 1983, the same group reported on an expanded analysis (Pike et al., 1983). There was a strong association with use of the pill before age 25: the relative risk was estimated to be 2.0 for four to six years of use and 4.9 for more than six years of use before age 25. The previous association with use before the first pregnancy was now attributed to a positive correlation between this variable and use before age 25. Attention was subsequently focused again on use before the first pregnancy by the results of a case-control study conducted in Britain by McPherson and colleagues (McPherson et al., 1983, 1987). They found a strong association with use before the first pregnancy but no effect of use after it—indeed, there was a suggestion that use occurring only after the first pregnancy might be protective.

Pike, McPherson, and Vessey were then instrumental in setting up the U.K. National Case-Control Study, with 755 cases under age 36 and an equal number of controls (U.K. National Case-Control Study Group, 1989). The results published in 1989 showed a highly significant trend in risk of breast cancer with total duration of pill use. But not only were the relative risk estimates much closer to 1.0 than in the previous studies; there was now no greater effect of use before the first pregnancy than after the first pregnancy. The results were presented clearly, but many readers apparently did not appreciate that the authors' previous hypothesis (about a risk confined to use at a specific time in early reproductive life) had been rejected.

Clearly, use before the first pregnancy, use before age 25, and total use will all be correlated, and many studies will have insufficient power to distinguish their effects with confidence. There is a danger, however, in focusing attention on the subgroup in each study that happens to give the highest relative risk estimate. This source of bias is illustrated by the summary table in a recent British review (Chilvers and Deacon, 1990), which shows only the subgroup in each study that gave the most positive results (ignoring the fact that negative results were obtained in some subgroups listed for other studies).

The second problem in interpreting recent findings is that in several of the best investigations, such as the U.K. National Study (U.K. National Case-Control Study Group, 1989), the relative risk estimates are close to 1.0. With relative risks of this order, epidemiologists find it difficult to exclude the possible influences of bias, confounding, and chance (Skegg, 1988). With regard to precautions taken to minimize and assess potential sources of bias, the U.K. National Study is the most adequate case-control study so far conducted; nevertheless, some problems remain. For example, selection (or nonresponse) bias is a possibility because only 72 percent of eligible cases could be interviewed (16 percent had died). Examination of general practice case-notes showed that the women with breast cancer who were not interviewed had, on average, significantly less oral contraceptive use than those who were interviewed. Data presented in the paper suggest that the relative risks should probably be scaled down by about 20 percent to allow for this bias, which would bring them even closer to 1.0.

The possibility of modification of the relative risk by confounding factors is always present in studies of this issue. Adjustments are made for known confounding variables but, because the main causes of breast cancer are unknown, unsuspected factors could be associated with both choosing oral contraception and the risk of developing breast cancer.

Cohort studies are free of some, although not all, of the sources of bias that can affect case-control studies, and definitive conclusions may be possible only with the completion of cohort studies containing large numbers of young women—such as the new Nurses' Health Study. The best synthesis of the evidence so far available from case-control and cohort studies is that oral contraceptives do produce a modest increase in the risk of developing breast cancer at a young age (up to about 35 years). This was the provisional conclusion reached by Sir Richard Doll, in summing up a recent conference at which data from most of the major studies were presented (Doll, 1990). Doll concluded that use of oral contraceptives produces no material increase in the risk of developing breast cancer after the age of about 45. With regard to the 35- to 44-year-old age group, he thought that it is "reasonable to postulate that there is some tailing off of the effect" occurring at younger ages.

AN EFFECT IN YOUNG WOMEN

If any adverse effect of oral contraceptives is confined to the risk of breast cancer developing at a young age, the situation is close to the more optimistic scenario considered by Vessey in his risk-benefit assessment (Vessey, 1990). Can it be confidently assumed, however, that the effect observed in young women will not extend in the future to the older ages at which breast cancer is common? It is essential to consider the possible explanations for the different results obtained recently in young and older women. Four possible explanations have differing implications for the future.

First, there could be a specific effect on the risk of breast cancer at a young age, which either tails off or reverses at older ages. This is the hypothesis advanced by Doll (1990), and it is plausible because there is known to be a "crossover" in the effects of some other risk factors for breast cancer with age (Janerich and Hoff, 1982; Ron et al., 1984).

Second, there could be an effect of recent use of the pill, which either tails off or reverses after some years. Here the best analogy would be with the initial influence of pregnancy. A full-term pregnancy appears to be followed by a short-term increase in the risk of breast cancer, which, after some years, is superseded by the protective effect of parity (Bruzzi et al., 1988). La Vecchia proposed that oral contraceptives might have an effect similar to that of pregnancy, although the evidence supporting this hypothesis is limited (La Vecchia, 1990).

Third, there could be an effect of use early in reproductive life, which has become common only among the most recent cohorts of women. This hypothesis led McPherson and others to suggest the possibility of a major epidemic of breast cancer as women in these cohorts age (McPherson et al., 1986). The results of the recent U.K. National Study provide no support for this explanation, because women who started using the pill at a young age (e.g., in their teens) were not found to be at higher risk than those who started later (U.K. National Case-Control Study Group, 1989). The final results from a large case-control study in New Zealand also provide evidence against an adverse effect of starting oral contraceptives before 20 years of age (Paul et al., 1990).

Fourth, there could be an effect of the particular formulations of the pill used by recent cohorts of women. Such an effect might also be expected to persist as these women move into older age groups. Again, the U.K. National Study provides no support for this explanation because relative risks were found to be higher for the older (high-estrogen) combined pills (U.K. National Case-Control Study Group, 1989). Nevertheless, it remains possible that some of the discrepancies among studies reflect geographic and temporal patterns of use of pills with particular steroid combinations or dosages.

Although doubt may persist until the present generation of young women moves into middle age and beyond, the first of these four explanations seems the most plausible at present.

CONCLUSIONS

All contraceptives cause breast cancer to the extent that delaying a woman's first pregnancy (and probably reducing her total number of pregnancies) increases her risk of breast cancer (Layde et al., 1989). The cloud hanging over oral contraceptives is the suggestion that these contraceptives may cause a specific increase in risk, at least in young women. The relationship between the pill and breast cancer appears complex and will not be clarified by a focus only on positive subgroups. If future studies are not to produce results that may be misleading from a public health viewpoint, they should cover the full range of ages of women who have used oral contraceptives (including women who have passed the menopause).

More research is needed before we can be certain that a risk of breast cancer does not outweigh the noncontraceptive benefits of oral contraception (especially in preventing ovarian cancer). Present evidence offers grounds for cautious optimism: breast cancer is not likely to tip the balance against oral contraceptives. The cloud over the pill may also have a silver lining if a better understanding of its relationship with breast cancer can lead to the design of hormonal contraceptives that reduce the risk of breast cancer, as well as cancers of the ovary and endometrium. The primary prevention of breast cancer will then be within our grasp.

REFERENCES

Bruzzi, P., E. Negri, C. La Vecchia, et al. 1988. Short-term increase in breast cancer risk following a full-term pregnancy. British Medical Journal 297:1096-1098.

Cancer and Steroid Hormone Study. 1987a. Combination oral contraceptive use and the risk of endometrial cancer. Journal of the American Medical Association 257:796-800.

Cancer and Steroid Hormone Study. 1987b. The reduction in risk of ovarian cancer associated with oral-contraceptive use. New England Journal of Medicine 316:650-655.

Chilvers, C. E. D., and J. M. Deacon. 1990. Oral contraceptives and breast cancer. British Journal of Cancer 61:1-4.

Contraception Report. 1990. Pp. 4-5 in The Media and Contraception, Vol. 1. Morris Plains, N.J.: Emron, Inc.

Doll, R. 1973. Monitoring the National Health Service. Proceedings of the Royal Society of Medicine 66:729-740.

Doll, R. 1990. What conclusions can we reach and how do we best assist women to make informed choices regarding their use of oral contraceptives? Pp. 395-400 in Oral Contraceptives and Breast Cancer, R. D. Mann, ed. Park Ridge, N.J.: Parthenon Publishing.

Forman, D., T. J. Vincent, and R. Doll. 1986. Cancer of the liver and the use of oral contraceptives. British Medical Journal 292:1357-1361.

Hulka, B. S. 1989. Hormonal contraceptives and risk of cervical cancer. Pp. 84-96 in Safety Requirements for Contraceptive Steroids, F. Michal, ed. Cambridge: Cambridge University Press.

Janerich, D. T., and M. B. Hoff. 1982. Evidence for a cross-over in breast cancer risk factors. American Journal of Epidemiology 116:737-742.

La Vecchia, C. 1990. Oral contraceptives and breast cancer: Update of an Italian case-control study. Pp. 245-251 in Oral Contraceptives and Breast Cancer, R. D. Mann, ed. Park Ridge, N.J.: Parthenon Publishing.

Layde, P. M., L. A. Webster, A. L. Baughman, et al. 1989. The independent associations of parity, age at first full term pregnancy, and duration of breastfeeding with the risk of breast cancer. Journal of Clinical Epidemiology 42:963-973.

Lund, E. 1989. Re: "Potential for bias in case-control studies of oral contraceptives and breast cancer" (letter). American Journal of Epidemiology 130:1066-1068.

Mann, R. D., ed. 1990. Oral Contraceptives and Breast Cancer. Park Ridge, N.J.: Parthenon Publishing.

McPherson, K., A. Neil, M. P. Vessey, and R. Doll. 1983. Oral contraceptives and breast cancer (letter). Lancet 2:1414-1415.

McPherson, K., P. A. Coope, and M. P. Vessey. 1986. Early oral contraceptive use and breast cancer: Theoretical effects of latency. Journal of Epidemiology and Community Health 40:289-294.

McPherson, K., M. P. Vessey, A. Neil, R. Doll, L. Jones, and M. Roberts. 1987. Early oral contraceptive use and breast cancer: Results of another case-control study. British Journal of Cancer 56:653-660.

Muir, C., J. Waterhouse, T. Mack, J. Powell, and S. Whelan, eds. 1987. Cancer Incidence in Five Continents, vol 5. Lyon: International Agency for Research on Cancer.

Neuberger, J., D. Forman, R. Doll, and R. Williams. 1986. Oral contraceptives and hepatocellular carcinoma. British Medical Journal 292:1355-1357.

Ory, H. W., J. D. Forrest, and R. Lincoln. 1983. Making choices: Evaluating the health risks and benefits of birth control methods. New York: Alan Guttmacher Institute.

Paul, C., D. C. G. Skegg, and G. F. S. Spears. 1990. Oral contraceptives and risk of breast cancer. International Journal of Cancer 46:366-373.

Pike, M. C., B. E. Henderson, J. T. Casagrande, I. Rosario, and G. E. Gray. 1981. Oral contraceptive use and early abortion as risk factors for breast cancer in young women. British Journal of Cancer 43:72-76.

Pike, M. C., B. E. Henderson, M. D. Krailo, A. Duke, and S. Roy. 1983. Breast cancer in young women and use of oral contraceptives: Possible modifying effect of formulation and age at use. Lancet 2:926-930.

Population Information Program. 1988. Lower-dose pills. Population Reports, Series A, No. 7. Johns Hopkins University, Baltimore, Md.

Potts, M., P. J. Feldblum, I. Chi, W. Liao, and A. Fuertes-de La Haba. 1982. The Puerto Rico oral contraceptive study: An evaluation of the methodology and results of a feasibility study. British Journal of Family Planning 7:99-103.

Prentice, R. L., and D. B. Thomas. 1987. On the epidemiology of oral contraceptives and disease. Advances in Cancer Research 49:285-401.

Ron, E., F. Lubin, and Y. Wax. 1984. Re: "Evidence for a cross-over in breast cancer risk factors" (letter). American Journal of Epidemiology 119:139-141.

Rooks, J. B., H. W. Ory, K. G. Ishak, et al. 1979. Epidemiology of hepatocellular adenoma. The role of oral contraceptive use. Journal of the American Medical Association 242:644-648.

Royston, E., and S. Armstrong, eds. 1989. Preventing Maternal Deaths. Geneva: World Health Organization.

Schlesselman, J. J. 1989. Cancer of the breast and reproductive tract in relation to use of oral contraceptives. Contraception 40:1-38.

Simonsen, J. N., F. A. Plummer, and E. N. Ngugi. 1990. HIV infection among lower socioeconomic strata prostitutes in Nairobi. AIDS 4:139-144.

Skegg, D. C. G. 1988. Potential for bias in case-control studies of oral contraceptives and breast cancer. American Journal of Epidemiology 127:205-212.

Stadel, B. V. 1981. Oral contraceptives and cardiovascular disease. New England Journal of Medicine 305:612-618, 672-677.

Swan, S. H., and D. B. Petitti. 1982. A review of the problems of bias and confounding in epidemiologic studies of cervical neoplasia and oral contraceptive use. American Journal of Epidemiology 115:10-18.

Thomas, D. B. 1989. The breast. Pp. 38-68 in Safety Requirements for Contraceptive Steroids, F. Michal, ed. Cambridge: Cambridge University Press.

Tietze, C., J. Bongaarts, and B. Schearer. 1976. Mortality associated with the control of fertility. Family Planning Perspectives 8:6-14.

U.K. National Case-Control Study Group. 1989. Oral contraceptive use and breast cancer risk in young women. Lancet 1:973-982.

Vessey, M. P. 1990. An overview of the benefits and risks of combined oral contraceptives. Pp. 121-132 in Oral Contraceptives and Breast Cancer, R. D. Mann, ed. Park Ridge, N.J.: Parthenon Publishing.

F

List of Background Documents

For this study, the Institute of Medicine invited and commissioned reports on various topics concerning oral contraceptives and breast cancer. Four of these reports appear in this volume (Appendixes A, B, D, and E). The manuscripts of eight other of these documents are available from the National Technical Information Service, 5285 Port Royal Road, Springfield, VA 22161; telephone 703-487-4650. NTIS document numbers are in parentheses.

"History of Oral Contraception," Richard A. Edgren, Director, Scientific Affairs, Syntex Laboratories, Inc., Palo Alto, Calif. (#PB91-186841)

"Safety of Oral Contraception," Richard A. Edgren, Director, Scientific Affairs, Syntex Laboratories, Inc., Palo Alto, Calif. (#PB91-186858)

"The Demographics of Oral Contraceptive Use," Jacqueline Darroch Forrest, Vice President for Research, The Alan Guttmacher Institute, New York, N.Y. (#PB91-186833)

"Hormone Effects on Biological Markers in Breast Cancer," Kenneth S. McCarty, Jr., and Kenneth S. McCarty, Sr., Departments of Biochemistry, Pathology, and Medicine, Duke University Medical Center, Durham, N.C. (#PB91-186825)

"Oral Contraceptives and Breast Cancer: A Review of the Epidemiological Evidence," Kathleen E. Malone, Department of Epidemiology, School of Public Health, University of Washington, Seattle, Wash. (Appendix A)

"Summary Table of Studies of Breast Cancer Risk Related to Oral Contraceptive Use (December 11, 1989)," Kathleen E. Malone, Department of Epidemiology, School of Public Health, University of Washington, Seattle, Wash. (#PB91-186973)

"Oral Contraceptives and Breast Cancer: Review of the Epidemiological Literature," David B. Thomas, Fred Hutchinson Cancer Research Center, University of Washington, Seattle, Wash. (Appendix B)

"Age-Specific Differences in the Relationship Between Oral Contraceptive Use and Breast Cancer," Phyllis A. Wingo, Nancy C. Lee, Howard W. Ory, Valerie Beral, Herbert B. Peterson, and P. Rhoades, Centers for Disease Control, Atlanta, Ga. (#PB91-186551)

"Animal Models of Sex Steroid Hormones and Mammary Cancer: Are There Lessons for Our Understanding of Studies in Humans?" Diana B. Petitti, Department of Family and Community Medicine, University of California School of Medicine, San Francisco, Calif. (Appendix D)

"Risks and Benefits of Oral Contraceptives: Will Breast Cancer Tip the Balance?" David C. G. Skegg, Department of Preventive and Social Medicine, University of Otago, Dunedin, New Zealand. (Appendix E)

"Oral Contraceptives and Breast Cancer: Issues Related to Age, Duration of Use, Dose, and Latent Effects," James J. Schlesselman, Department of Preventive Medicine and Biometrics, School of Medicine, Uniformed Services University of the Health Sciences, Bethesda, Md. (#PB91-186569)

"Modeling Risks and Benefits of Oral Contraceptives," Judith Fortney and Michele Bonhomme, Division of Reproductive Epidemiology and Sexually Transmitted Diseases, Family Health International, Research Triangle Park, N.C. (#PB91-186817)

Index

177